GW01398728

The Natural Skin Care

PLAYBOOK

EVERYTHING YOU NEED TO KNOW ABOUT PLANT-BASED BEAUTY

The Natural Skin Care PLAYBOOK

DR. CHRISTINA HECTOR

publish your gift

THE NATURAL SKIN CARE PLAYBOOK

Published by Publish Your Gift®

An imprint of Purposely Created Publishing Group, LLC

Printed in the United States of America

ISBN: 978-1-64484-595-0 (print)

ISBN: 978-1-64484-596-7 (ebook)

Dedication

This book is dedicated to my loving husband who always supports my creative ideas.

Table of Contents

Introduction

My journey to creating skin care products started in medical school. It may have been the stress from studying or the lack of time for self-care, but I began to see a change in my hair. My hair became weak, thin, damaged, and I did not know how to fix it. So, I searched for a hairstylist who could help restore my damaged hair. By the time I reached the third hairstylist, I was convinced that she could help restore the health of my hair.

After a few months of going to my new hairstylist, she pointed out my hair's poor health. However, when I asked her what I should do to fix the problem, she could not provide any solutions. I became discouraged. Not wanting to look for a fourth hairstylist, I had to admit to myself the root cause of my problem: the chemicals I had applied to my hair for the previous sixteen years.

While in medical school, I was more aware of the information coming to the surface about the harmful ingredients found in hair care products. Performing my research,

I learned that these chemical products could also harm my overall health and wellness. It became apparent that if I did not stop using chemicals in my hair, I would have irreversible hair and scalp damage. Scarier was the possibility of developing health issues due to these chemicals. I knew I had to find a solution.

The solution to this problem was to stop using chemicals in my hair and cut off all damaged hair. However, I was not sure if I was ready for that transformation. So, I made another trip to the hairstylist. My hairstylist was friendly, direct, and full of stories. She was a nice escape from my medical school studies. Then she asked one question, and I knew this would be my last visit to see her. "What are you doing to your hair?" I did not give her an answer. I went home after my appointment, vowing that this would be the last chemical placement in my hair.

The next step was deciding how I would transition my hair from chemically processed to natural—having natural hair meant keeping my hair in its natural state without using chemicals. My continued research landed me on YouTube. On YouTube, there were women with similar problems and similar solutions. I remember lying on my living room couch with the laptop in front of me until 3:00 a.m. absorbing all the information available. By the time I was ready for bed, I had finalized my plans to transition my hair from chemically processed to natural hair.

In this transformation, I cut off all my chemically processed hair. Then I had to change all of my hair care products. That included the shampoo, conditioner, oils, and styling products. Although I became more vigilant about the ingredients listed on hair care products, I soon realized few natural hair products were available. If I did find a product, it was too expensive for my medical school budget. I became frustrated. I often walked into a beauty supply store only to walk out empty-handed.

I went through many products during my family medicine residency years. When I started my sports medicine fellowship, I was closer to narrowing down my hair care products. However, I was not 100 percent satisfied with the products I purchased. During this time, I had the creative idea to make hair care products using only natural ingredients I had already researched over the years.

For the first time in a long time, I was happy with the products I used in my hair, not only because they were my products, but also because my hair was thick, shiny, and healthy. I could not stop at hair care products. Many synthetic ingredients in commercial hair care products are also in daily skin care products. I soon started to create skin care products. The summer after completing my sports medicine fellowship, I gradually transitioned out every skin care product in my house to natural products I formulated and produced.

[illegible] went through many products [illegible] during my many med[illegible] [illegible] years. When I started my [illegible] prints, [illegible] was close to [illegible] down [illegible] [illegible]

[illegible] products using only natural [illegible] already used [illegible] drying [illegible]

[illegible] first time in a long time, I was happy with the products I used on my [illegible], not only [illegible] [illegible]

Chapter 1

Skin Care: The Past, Regulations, and Business of Skin Care

A BRIEF HISTORY OF SKIN CARE

Skin care regimens date back to ancient Egypt. During this era, the ancient Egyptians used olive oil and natural clay mixtures for cleansing the skin, milk masks to moisturize the skin, and dead sea salts as an exfoliant.[1] Their skin care included natural plant ingredients such as chamomile, rosemary, and lavender.[2] It also contained pressed oil from the seeds of the castor, sesame, and moringa plant. In addition, the Egyptians' makeup served "to help decorate their skin and also to protect them from the harsh elements of the sun and desert."[3] The making of skin care products moved into ancient Greece, where treatments for anti-aging skin used ingredients such as olive oil, honey, milk, and yogurt.

In India, over five thousand years ago, Ayurvedic herbs were discovered and used for their holistic and medicinal properties. They provide the body with the balance it needs to help prevent illness and maintain health; this includes restoring and maintaining the health of the skin and hair. Ayurveda herbs are also becoming well-known for their skin and hair benefits and are part of the new studies for cosmeceutical products.

In the United States during the 1800s, skin care products were mainly made by women at home. They used natural ingredients to beautify the skin by making it "smoother, cleaner, whiter, clearer, and glowing."[4] In addition, their skin care products were also known to contain medicinal properties that helped to "remove freckles and ruddiness, to calm rashes, or to reverse the damage done by wind and sunburn."[5] These products came from recipes shared amongst mothers, family members, and friends.

In the 1900s, there was an explosion of skin care products in the US. No longer were skin care products made at home, passed down through generations, or only shared with family and friends. In this era, there was a mass movement to sell skin care products to the masses. With this came the manufacturing factories and retail stores. It was the birth of many skin care businesses, with many of those businesses still existing today.

There is not much difference between the eighteenth century and the twenty-first centuries as more people seek natural properties in their skin care. Consumers want their skin care to benefit, heal, and protect their skin. The skin care industry evolved from women making products at home to mass manufacturing, back to women starting skin care companies in their homes.

THE WOMEN PIONEERS OF SKIN CARE

The skin care industry started to take rise in the US in the nineteenth century. Taking the lead were women who took their at-home creations and sold them to the people. For example, in 1889, Anne Malone developed hair and scalp products. She sold her products door-to-door in the beginning and hired women to sell her products for her. She then moved on to open her first storefront in 1904 and further on to opening Poro College in 1918.[6] Anne Malone became "the first commercially available black skin care founder and one of the first black millionaires."[7] She set the framework for black women to follow.

Attending Ann Malone's school was Madam C. J. Walker. Under Malone, Walker perfected her hair care products, and in 1905 she started selling her scalp products door-to-door throughout the south. In 1908, Madam C. J. Walker opened a factory and a beauty school in Pittsburg; in 1910, Madam C. J. Walker transferred her manufacturing company to Indianapolis, where she manufactured and sold her own line of hair and skin care products.[8]

The skin care industry continues to evolve and now becomes sold in "upscale, brand-dedicated shops, in druggists and department stores, or by licensed agents."[9] In 1910,

Elizabeth Arden opened her first store in New York. Elizabeth Arden, originally from Canada, started her beauty industry journey in nursing school. Then, she moved to New York and worked in a beauty salon. In 1910, she opened her first salon store. Her interest in creams and lotions propelled her to continue to grow her brand by working with chemists to develop her line of creams.

Estée Lauder was one of the first to sell her cosmetic products at Saks Fifth Avenue. The Estée Lauder brand was founded in 1946 after Estée Lauder learned the business from her chemist uncle. She started with the sale of "cold cream, lip rouge, and fragrances. Estée Lauder cosmetics were sold primarily at department stores."[10] In 1963, Mary Kay Ash founded Beauty by Mary Kay. She sold products using the direct sale model of door-to-door. The company became known for its signature pink and the name shortened to Mary Kay.

THE REGULATIONS IN THE SKIN CARE INDUSTRY

Many of these beauty company names and products continue to thrive well into the twenty-first century. As the industry grew, so did the need for regulation due to the boom of potential profits from selling beauty products. Unfortunately, many products advertised in the market did not have the beneficial values stated on the products. Some of the products even posed potential harm. As a result, people became concerned about these products and their lack of regulation. It was not until 1937, when "one company marketed a new 'wonder drug' to treat strep infection (usually in children), which included a chemical compound similar to antifreeze,"[11] that Congress moved for more regulation. In this tragic event, "over one hundred people died from the medicine."[12] Soon after, in 1938, Congress passed the Federal Food, Drug, and Cosmetic Act.

The Federal Food, Drug, and Cosmetic Act (FD&C Act) describes a cosmetic as an "article intended to be rubbed, poured, sprinkled, or sprayed on, introduced into, or otherwise applied to the human body."[13] This application is either for "cleansing, beautifying, promoting attractiveness, or altering the appearance."[14] The cosmetic regulations include "moisturizers, perfumes, lipsticks, nail polish, most make-up, and shampoos."[15] Under these regulations, products that state to have a medicinal property are classified as a drug and not a cosmetic. For example, "a regular shampoo would be classified as a cosmetic, but an anti-dandruff shampoo would be a drug."[16]

The Food and Drug Administration (FDA) is the regulator of the cosmetic industry. However, their legal authority over cosmetics differs from that of other regulated products such as drugs, biologics, and medical devices. For instance, the FDA does not require cosmetic products and ingredients other than color additives to gain the FDA's approval before going on the market. However, there are some laws and regulations in place that apply to cosmetics on the market.

The FD&C Act prohibits the marketing of adulterated or misbranded products. "Adulteration" refers to violations involving product composition, whether from ingredients, contaminants, processing, packaging, or shipping and handling.[17] "Misbranding" refers to violations involving improperly labeled or deceptively packaged products.[18]

The second law is the Fair Packaging and Labeling Act (FPLA), which does not allow unfair or deceptive packaging or labeling. Each packaging must contain the following:

- A statement identifying the product
- The name and place of business of the manufacturer, packer, or distributor
- The net quantity of contents in terms of weight, measure, or numerical count (measurement must be in both metric and imperial units)

However, the fact remains that cosmetics do not have to receive FDA approval before going on the market. Due to this, harmful ingredients can make their way into our skin care products. Even with the FDA regulations, reports have surfaced on the toxic ingredients in some commercial skin care products, which we will discuss further in this book.

THE DISCOVERY OF SOAP

The history of soap dates as far back as ancient Babylon, where archeologists found remnants of soap-like material in clay cylinders; these cylinders contained inscriptions that we understand to mean "fats boiled with ashes," a soapmaking method.[19] In ancient Egypt, combining animal fats and vegetable oils with alkaline salts would form soap-like material used for washing and treating skin disease.[20]

Legend says that soap was named after Mount Sapo in ancient Rome, where the melted fat from animals sacrificed on top of the mountain would mix with wood ashes, forming a clay mixture that made cleaning easier. Soapmaking traveled throughout Italy, Spain, and France due to their ready supplies of source ingredients, such as oil from olive trees.

In the nineteenth century, soapmaking became one of America's fastest-growing industries. One of the first commercially sold floating soaps was the Ivory soap, invented in 1878 by James N. Gamble and his business partner, Harley Procter.

This process of soapmaking continued until the twentieth century. However, during World War I and World War II, there were shortages in the animal fats and vegetable oils that were used for soap making. Instead, synthetic chemicals with similar properties replaced soap. These are what are known today as "detergents."[21]

IS IT A SOAP OR IS IT A DETERGENT?

The question of whether a soap is a true soap or a detergent dictates how it is regulated. While cosmetics are regulated by the FDA, true soap is not. Traditional soap is produced using animal fats, known as tallow or lard, or plant-based oil. To make a traditional soap, you will need to combine the animal fat or the plant-based oil with an alkali. An alkali is a chemical base with a pH of seven. The alkali used for soapmaking is commonly known as lye.

In the process of soapmaking, the fatty particles of the fat or oil break down and interact with the lye to make soap—a process called saponification. If the soap is made correctly, there is no more lye left in the product and you are left with a cleanser, the soap. A true soap cannot be made without an alkali.

I learned this very early on in my research on how to make natural soap. At first, learning about lye turned me away from wanting to make soap. I started to look for no-lye soapmaking recipes; however, with more research, I made two observations. Either the lye process was previously performed in the no-lye soap base, or the no-lye soap base contained synthetic ingredients, making it a detergent and not a soap. I wanted to make true soap.

Many of the soaps we are using now are not true soaps. They are actually synthetic detergents.

Based on the FDA regulations, there are three criteria for a true (traditional) soap:

1. The product produced must be made with an animal fat or plant-based oil and alkali.
2. The finished product from the combination of animal fat/plant-based oil and alkali must be the main cleaning ingredient of the soap. If the product has synthetic ingredients used for cleansing, it is a cosmetic, not a soap.
3. The many properties of soap are for cleansing. The soap cannot have any additional properties such as making you smell good (that's a cosmetic) or antibacterial properties (that will make the product a drug and it will be regulated differently per the FDA).

Interestingly, even if the product per the FDA regulation is a synthetic detergent, a cosmetic, or a drug, the product can still be called soap. This name play can be confusing to the mass public. If you walk down the "soap" aisle in a supermarket, there are no labels designating body detergents. They state soap. However, the products do not meet the three regulatory criteria to be a true (traditional) soap.

With that said, true soap is not regulated by the FDA. Instead, it is regulated by the Consumer Product Safety

Commission (CPSC). The CPSC's purpose is to protect the public from unreasonable risks of injury or death associated with consumer products under its jurisdiction.[22] The FDA continues to regulate cleansing products not classified as true (traditional) soap.

THE REGULATION OF NEWER TERMS

Natural skin care is generally defined as products made with ingredients found in nature. Under the FDA regulation, there is no set definition for "natural." Natural skin care products will fall under the same requirements of the Federal Food, Drug, and Cosmetic Act and the Fair Packaging and Labeling Act. These FDA regulations hold whether the product ingredients are plant, animal, mineral, or synthetic.

A bill that has yet to pass is the Natural Cosmetics Act; its purpose is to define and regulate the word "natural" in skin care products as to not be misleading to the consumer. The Natural Cosmetics Act describes "the term 'natural' as 'any chemical substance that is naturally occurring and which is (i) unprocessed; (ii) processed only by manual, mechanical, naturally derived solvent or gravitational means, by dissolution in water or steam, by flotation, or by heating solely to remove water; or (iii) extracted from air by any means."[23] I do believe that in the years to come the term "natural," or any additional labels placed on skin care products including cosmetics, will have a more precise definition for skin care companies to stay true to their messaging and for consumer safety and transparency. Currently, the FDA guidelines on cosmetics have not changed in over eighty years. The FDA does not regulate the term "natural."

Organic skin care products are regulated by the National Organic Program (NOP), which is overseen by the US Department of Agriculture (USDA). The NOP "develops and enforces consistent national standards" amongst the organic agricultural products made in the US.[24] It also regulates the ingredient labels to assure that the percentage of organic ingredients listed on the label meets the national standard. Many skin care products contain the label "organic" or state that they are made with organic ingredients. However, it is unknown whether the product meets all the standards without the USDA stamp.

An organic skin care product will have to follow the USDA requirements for the use of the term "organic" and will also have to follow the FDA regulation for cosmetics. Therefore, we can assume that if the product is an organic "true" soap, it will follow the USDA and CPSC requirements.

Dr. Albert Kligman developed he term "cosmeceuticals" in 1984. A cosmeceutical is the fusion of a cosmetic and a pharmaceutical. Dr. Kligman defines it as "a topical preparation that is sold as a cosmetic but has performance characteristics that suggest pharmaceutical action."[25] Currently, the Federal Food, Drug, and Cosmetic Act does not recognize this as a category. Per the FD&C Act, "a product can be a drug, a cosmetic, or a combination of both; however, the actual term 'cosmeceuticals' has no meaning under the law."[26]

Clean beauty is, as of now, the newest term to hit the market and continues to grow as the market looks for products with fewer chemicals. What is now noticed is the lack of regulation of cosmetic products by the FDA as compared to other countries around the world. This lack of regulation leads to skin care products with harmful chemicals that can increase cancer risk, congenital disabilities, and reproductive complications.

THE BUSINESS OF SKIN CARE

The ever-growing industry of skin care is fascinating. The skin care industry never fails to continue its growth and reinvent itself; this makes skin care the largest percentage of the American cosmetics and hygiene industry. The global skin care product market was worth about $140.92 billion in 2020. It is predicted to grow at a compound annual growth rate (CAGR) of 4.69 percent by 2026.[27]

The natural skin care industry, just a piece of the whole skin care industry, has continued to grow, gaining traction from people looking for an alternative to the synthetic and chemical ingredients found in most commercial skin care products. Based on a report published by Grand View

Research, Inc., "The global natural cosmetics market size is expected to reach a value of USD 48.04 billion by 2025, at a CAGR of 5.01 percent from 2019 to 2025. High demand for natural health and wellness products among millennials due to increasing awareness about the harmful impact of synthetic chemicals is driving the growth."[28]

Skin care is a necessity, as indicated by the market growth. Daily we are at least using a type of moisturizer, or a lip product, or a cleansing product. We, the consumers, are always searching for the "it" product that will decrease or eliminate our skin flaws. We will always look for products that will provide us with youthful skin, as you can see with the ever-growing skin care industry that has to continue to deliver these products.

Today, using products just for a youthful look is not enough. Consumers are looking for properties in skin care that benefit, heal, and protect their skin. Consumers are also looking for products that do not use harmful ingredients, do not pollute the world, and are kind to animals. These criteria are part of the growing shift to natural skin care products.

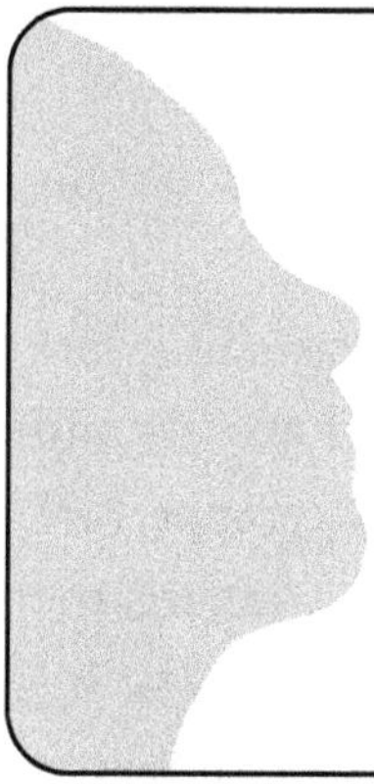

Chapter 2

Skin Care Starts at the Anatomy and Ends at the Ingredients

THE HUMAN SKIN

Did you know that the human skin is an organ? In fact, it is the largest organ of the human body. It has a multitude of complex functions. First, let me put on my doctor's coat to talk about the anatomy of the skin, as it is essential to understand further the importance of being selective when choosing the products to put on your skin.

The skin consists of three layers of specialized cells and structures: the epidermis, dermis, and the hypodermis. Each layer has its specific function. The epidermis is the outermost layer of the skin. It serves as a barrier to water, which prevents it from seeping through the skin and entering the body. This layer of skin is the first line of defense against the invasion of microorganisms that cause infections. The epidermis is also a mechanical and chemical barrier to trauma and damage from ultraviolet (UV) light.[29]

The next layer is called the dermis. It consists of layers of fat and connective tissue containing blood vessels and nerves. The dermis is vital for skin and body temperature regulations. It is also the area of the skin that contains the hair follicles, sweat glands, and sebaceous glands.[30] The innermost layer of the skin is the hypodermis, also known as the subcutaneous connective tissue. It contains adipose tissue composed of fat cells, sensory neurons, blood vessels, and some skin appendages.

The general appearance, turgor, and other qualities of the skin can also give insight into the general health of the body. Skin that is dry, dull, and brittle can easily crack, causing microorganisms to enter and leading to infections of the skin and the body. Dry skin loses moisture, causing rashes and scaly skin as it tries to repair itself from micro-injuries. Dry skin can experience an increase in wrinkles and age spots and can appear dull with little care. If your skin has a poorly functioning epidermis, it may not synthesize vitamin D properly, causing an increased insult to the skin from UV light from the sun. Severely damaged skin will try to heal by forming scar tissue. These scar tissues are often discolored and depigmented. Wrinkles are caused by a breakdown of the collagen and elastin within the dermis, which results in sagging skin.

The skin is also a target for oxidative stress. Oxidative stress happens when there is an imbalance between the skin's reactive oxygen species (free radicals) and the body's defense mechanisms. Free radicals are an unstable chemical species with an unpaired electron. Having an unpaired electron forces the chemical species to search and take an electron from a stable atom or molecule of a cell. Losing an electron causes damage to that cell. These free radicals are either intrinsic—a byproduct made in our body—or extrinsic from sources such as UV radiation, alcohol intake, poor nutrition, overeating, and severe physical and psychological stressors.[31]

Antioxidants are what we call the scavengers of free radicals. Antioxidants help to stabilize these free radicals, preventing them from causing cell damage. The human body's cells produce the antioxidants needed to help maintain cellular health, such as alpha lipoic acid and glutathione. There are likely many more undiscovered antioxidants made by the body's cells. The studies are ongoing. Research is also continuing on the plants containing antioxidants that are beneficial to the human body, and in particular, to the skin cells.

THE HEALING POWER OF PLANTS

Plants became known during ancient times and throughout the centuries for their ability to heal ailments, including skin ailments. This ability is due to the natural chemicals in plants called phytomolecules. This chemical compound contains many antioxidant properties. Some of the antioxidant properties included in phytomolecules are "flavonoids, tocopherols, carotenoids, phenols, betacarotene, lycopene, sesamol, gossypol, anthocyanins, catechins, ellagic acid, lutein, resveratrol, cinnamic acids, benzoic acids, folic acid, ascorbic acid, and tocotrienols."[32] They can scavenge free radical formations, helping our skin cells prevent disorders and cell damage.

There are many ways our body can benefit from the healing power of plants. As we know, plants are used to make teas. We mainly drink teas; however, teas can be used as a rinse for our hair or a soak for the skin and body relaxation. Herbs from plants can be infused in oils and added to ointments, salves, and lotions or used as a massage oil. Seeds from plants are expressed to make the cooking and body oils we use today. Plant kernels are used to make different kinds of butter. We cannot leave out essential oils, which are concentrated plant molecules extracted by steam distillation.

I recommend seeking medical attention for specific skin conditions. However, I also believe we need to focus on maintaining the skin's homogeneity, ensuring we are feeding it beneficial ingredients, and aiding the skin in performing its functions to the best of its ability. The point when our skin cannot perform its normal functions properly is when we develop dry skin, rashes, discoloration, sensitive skin, itchy skin, or scaly skin.

Think about it this way. If you have an illness, your doctor will provide a treatment—this can be a medication with specific properties to treat your condition. However, the doctor will still recommend eating healthy, drinking water, exercising, and taking vitamins as a way to maintain your health. This recommendation also holds for the skin, as we have to maintain the health of our skin.

SYNTHETIC INGREDIENTS IN SKIN CARE

Chemists create synthetic ingredients in a laboratory. First, they study the plant's properties down to the key molecules. Then, these molecules are further analyzed to make synthetic versions that mimic the plant's beneficial properties. Research continues even today as chemists continue to make synthetic products to fit the demands for more youthful skin.

Synthetic ingredients have the capability of being mass-produced. One reason is their stability. They are not affected by natural elements such as the weather since they are made in a laboratory. However, harsh weather or disasters can affect the supply of plant ingredients needed to manufacture skin care products. Also, synthetic ingredients are inexpensive to produce compared to cultivating and harvesting plant ingredients.

Another benefit for companies using synthetic products is their long shelf life. For example, skin care products with natural ingredients have shelf lives ranging from six months to a year. In contrast, skin care products with synthetic ingredients have shelf lives ranging from one to two years, essentially making them a more stable product.

These skin care products are known as commercial skin care products. These are the products commonly found on store shelves. They consist of your everyday skin care products such as lotion, shampoo, conditioner, and soap, to name a few. Commercial skin care products are made of mainly synthetic compounds and chemical ingredients.

In the latter half of the twentieth century, studies showed adverse effects and health concerns regarding some synthetic ingredients in skin care products. Some chemicals used in many skin care and cosmetic products can cause undesirable side effects, especially for people with sensitive skin and potential allergic reactions.[33] These revealing studies created a need to reevaluate these ingredients while also causing a shift for people to look for more natural products.

Here is a list of synthetic ingredients in skin care products that caused concerns:

Phthalate – Phthalate is a plastic additive found in many products we use, including skin care. Phthalates are in commercial skin care products such as moisturizers, lotions, shampoos, conditioners, and hair sprays, to name a few. The term "phthalate" is often not listed; instead, it is either not labeled or disguised as a fragrance. Although some scientists state that a small amount of phthalate is harmless, many studies have shown that phthalates can be absorbed in the body and potentially cause adverse effects on the endocrine system. The endocrine system regulates the body's hormones. Phthalates can disrupt this regulation, causing adverse effects on the reproductive, neurological, and developmental hormonal pathways. These potential effects are especially detrimental to children if exposed to phthalates at higher levels. Countries in the European Union have banned phthalates in skin care products. Currently, the FDA states that there is no harm in using of phthalates in skin care products. Although phthalate use has decreased over the years, there are no bans in the United States.

Paraben – Parabens are a group of chemicals used as preservatives in skin care products. They help to decrease the formation of bacteria, mold, and yeast in skin care products, particularly products with higher water content. Parabens also extend their shelf lives. Commercial products such as moisturizers, makeup, and hair care products often contain paraben. Scientific studies show that parabens can disrupt the reproductive organs by affecting fertility and increasing the risk of miscarriage. They can also increase the risk of cancer. Currently, the FDA has no restrictions on using parabens in cosmetic products. Five parabens have been completely banned in the EU (isopropylparaben, isobutylparaben, phenylparaben, benzylparaben, and pentylparaben), while others are strictly regulated because they are believed to be endocrine disruptors. In addition, the intergovernmental Association of Southeast Asian Nations (ASEAN) has also banned ten parabens in Southeast Asian countries.[34]

However, changes are slower in the US. Per the CDC, the "human health effects from environmental exposure to low levels of parabens are unknown. In 2006, the industry-led Cosmetic Ingredient Review (CIR), in a partnership with the US Food and Drug Administration (FDA), determined that there was no need to change CIR's original conclusion from 1984 that parabens are safe for use in cosmetics."[35] With this conclusion, the FDA continues to allow the addition of parabens to food sources as a means to preserve the food. However, many major stores across the US are banning products containing parabens from their shelves. Whole Foods Market has banned at least four parabens from the skin care collections featured in the stores. CVS has banned paraben in its line of beauty and personal care products for adults and babies. However, no bans on non-CVS items in their stores. Target has placed similar prohibitions. Also following suit are Walgreens and Rite Aid.

Preservatives "help prevent the growth of mold and fungus in cosmetic products. Because consumer preferences are shifting away from parabens, the FDA currently prioritizes enforcement against cosmetics that claim to use 'natural preservatives' or 'no preservatives' over traditional cosmetics because of the concern about the growth of bacteria."[36] However, as you continue to read through this book, you will find that there are ways to preserve cosmetic products without using harmful ingredients.

Formaldehyde-Releasing Preservatives – Formaldehyde is a preservative that prevents spoilage and the formation of bacteria and fungus in cosmetic products. Using it extends the product's shelf life. Formaldehyde-releasing preservatives work by releasing "a small amount of formaldehyde over time to preserve the product; this is known as 'off-gassing.'" The off-gassing of formaldehyde is a concern, as inhalation can lead to potential health risks.[37]

Formaldehyde is found in commonly used products such as nail polish, hair straightener, and hair dye. It has also been found in some baby shampoos and soaps.[38] With this said, the EU banned formaldehyde from beauty products in Europe. In the US, many stores such as Whole Foods, CVS, and Target also ban the sale of formaldehyde products. However, some skin care companies are using formaldehyde-producing chemicals in skin care products or disguising formaldehyde as a fragrance.

Fragrances – Fragrance is a synthetic ingredient that gives a scent to a product. It can be a unique scent, like in a perfume, a replicated scent that we are familiar with, such as key lime pie, or it can replicate an essential oil scent. Fragrances are ingredients often used in skin care products. Many chemicals used in skin care products disguise themselves as "fragrance."

Butylated hydroxyanisole (BHA) and butylated hydroxytoluene (BHT) – These were introduced in food and cosmetic products in the 1940s. They are synthetic antioxidants used for the preservation and extension of shelf life. These products include lipsticks, moisturizers, and creams. Based on the research done by the International Agency for Research on Cancer, BHA is classified as a possible human carcinogen. Additional concerns about BHA and BHT are that they can potentially mimic estrogen, causing reproductive harm, skin irritation, and allergic reactions.[39]

Bans have been placed on BHA in Europe and California due to their possible cancer-causing properties. In addition, the labeling of BHA can be confusing. For example, beta hydroxy acid is "commonly used in exfoliant and anti-aging products."[40] Beta hydroxy acid is also known as salicylic acid, which can increase sensitivity to sunlight; however, this product is currently considered safe by the FDA.

Coal Tar Dyes – Coal tar dyes were often found in hair dyes and shampoos. This product is a known carcinogen;

however, studies are mixed on its harmful effects when used as a hair dye. Currently, in Canada, "some coal tar dyes are prohibited in products that are used in the eye (like eyeshadow and mascara) but are allowed in hair dyes."[41] There are different rules in the US for the use of coal tar dye in hair dye. The FDA outlines these regulations requiring specific warning labels on hair dye products.

Dioxane – You may not have heard of dioxane as it is often not listed on ingredients lists. Dioxan is "found in many liquid products that create suds like shampoo, hand soap, bubble baths, and liquid soaps."[42] Research on dioxane show that it's a possible carcinogen and can affect the breast tissue. Dioxan is listed by the Environmental Protection Agency (EPA) as a carcinogen. It is currently not listed as a cosmetic ingredient by the FDA because it is considered a "manufacturing by-product," making dioxane very prevalent in common household products and cosmetics.[43]

Ethanolamines (DEA, MEA, TEA, and Related Chemicals) – One concern with synthetic products is that because they are chemicals, there is always a possibility of chemicals reacting with other chemicals, causing adverse effects. DEA is a synthetic ingredient that creates creamy or sudsy consistency in cosmetic products. When DEA reacts with the nitrites found in cosmetic products, the reaction produces nitrosamines, "a known human carcinogen."[44] Due to this possible chemical reaction, "the European Union restricts the use of DEA in cosmetics. It also limits the maximum concentration of nitrosamine produced containing these ingredients."[45]

Triclosan – Many products such as hand soaps and hand sanitizers contain the antibacterial chemical triclosan. Also, "a wide range of household products, including garbage bags, toys, linens, mattresses, toilet fixtures, clothing, furniture fabric, paints, and laundry detergent," contain triclosan.[46] The concern with triclosan is that it can be absorbed through the skin, not only having the ability to irritate the skin but also possibly being a human endocrine disruptor. In studies by the US Center for Disease Control and Prevention, "scientists detected triclosan in the urine of nearly 75 percent of those tested (2,517 people ages six years and older)."[47] Due to triclosan's long half-life, it takes longer to break down, damaging aquatic wildlife. With these findings, the FDA "issued regulations finding that triclosan and triclocarbon, along with twenty-three other chemicals, were no longer generally recognized as safe and effective when used in over-the-counter hand washes."[48]

Talc – Talc powder became a concern in a Johnson and Johnson lawsuit for claims that talc powder causes ovarian cancer. Talc is often in baby powders and other products, such as cosmetic powder, blushes, and eyeshadows. The Johnson and Johnson lawsuit claimed that the "lifelong use of baby powder caused ovarian cancer in some women," with additional lawsuits claiming that "talc powder contained trace amounts of asbestos."[49] There is no certainty if talc powder itself was the source or if it was an additional product ingredient. Further studies found "no association between talc use and ovarian cancer."[50]

There have been debates about the studies performed on the harmful effects of these discussed ingredients. However, another side to this discussion. "Some scientific articles suggest that the current method of testing ingredients (high dose studies on simulated skin or animals and creating a dose-response curve) is insufficient to show the true risk from lower levels of exposure."[51] Other studies state that the makeup of these different chemicals breaks down in the body differently and that using products containing multiple chemicals has few cumulative effects. Also, studies consider the dose-effect—how much of the chemical needs to be absorbed to cause a harmful effect? These studies state that the dose of the chemicals is so small that "it is unlikely that long-term use of cosmetics can have a harmful effect."[52]

No substantial evidence shows how much the body absorbs cosmetics with routine use. In some studies, it can be challenging to decipher the exact cancer-causing exposure since environmental factors also play a role and many studies take years to complete. Per the American Cancer Society, "because it is difficult to do long-term studies, there is virtually no information available about the long-term health effects of cosmetic use."[53]

The question remains, if there is a change in harm to the people using the products containing these potentially harmful ingredients, why incorporate them into the products? Are there alternative options where we do not have to question safety? Nonetheless, many countries have taken the stance to eliminate the use of harmful substances in skin care. The European Union (EU), containing twenty-seven countries, established its ban on harmful ingredients that can be linked to "cancer and birth defects regardless of the concentration of the chemical" in the product.[54]

The European Union Cosmetic Directive (76/768/EEC) was implemented in **January 2003** and updated in 2013 as the European Commission Regulation 1223/2009. This law banned "over 1,400 chemicals from cosmetics that are known or suspected to cause cancer, genetic mutation, reproductive harm or birth defects" are banned.[55] As of March 1, 2022, more chemicals have been added to the list.

Although the FDA does not have nearly the same amount of chemicals banned for use in cosmetic ingredients, many individual states are passing legislation to ban certain harmful substances. California's Toxic-Free Cosmetics Act (Assembly Bill 2762) will "prohibit a person or entity from manufacturing, selling, delivering, holding, or offering for sale, in commerce any cosmetic product that contains any of several specified intentionally added ingredients, except under specified circumstances."[56] This bill will commence on January 1, 2025. The passing of this bill will make California the first to establish a state-level band of twenty-four ingredients from beauty and personal care products.[57]

The ingredients included are:

1. Dibutyl phthalate
2. Diethylhexyl phthalate
3. Formaldehyde
4. Paraformaldehyde
5. Methylene glycol
6. Quaternium-15
7. Mercury
8. Isobutylparaben
9. Isopropylparaben
10. m-Phenylenediamine and its salts
11. o-Phenylenediamine and its salts
12. The following per- and polyfluoroalkyl substances (PFAS) and their salts:
    A. Perfluorooctane sulfonate (PFOS); heptadecafluorooctane-1-sulfonic acid

B. Potassium perfluorooctanesulfonate; potassium heptadecafluorooctane-1-sulfonate
C. Diethanolamine perfluorooctane sulfonate
D. Ammonium perfluorooctane sulfonate; ammonium heptadecafluorooctanesulfonate
E. Lithium perfluorooctane sulfonate; lithium heptadecafluorooctanesulfonate
F. Perfluorooctanoic acid (PFOA)
G. Ammonium pentadecafluorooctanoate
H. Nonadecafluorodecanoic acid
I. Ammonium nonadecafluorodecanoate
J. Sodium nonadecafluorodecanoate
K. Perfluorononanoic acid (PFNA)
L. Sodium heptadecafluorononanoate
M. Ammonium perfluorononanoate[47]

Because these harmful and dangerous chemicals are so prevalent in today's manufactured skin care products, the only safe solution is to experiment with natural and organic skin care products, whether that is through purchasing or making your own (to be discussed in the next section) until you find the right products that are beneficial and nonhazardous to your health.

WHAT ARE NATURAL SKIN CARE PRODUCTS?

Natural skin care products are plant-based products. Using plant-based products for your skin and health is not a new concept. The skin was traditionally treated with plants before modern medications. Plants in many different forms, including "teas, infusions, decoctions, ointments, and creams," served to moisturize the skin, treat wounds, and soothe rashes.[58] It was the primary way to treat illness and care for the skin. In the twenty-first century, a resurgence of natural skin care came after many reports of the potential harm of certain chemicals and synthetically made commercial skin care products. Customers are looking for products with health benefits, not products that can potentially cause harm.

The word "natural" in skin care products generally means "not synthetic" or "not made in the lab." The FDA does not have an official definition of the word "natural" as it pertains to skin care. They generally state natural products as "not containing chemically synthesized molecules, assuring a gentle action on the skin, coming from an ecologically friendly production process, or produced by an animal-testing-free process. We define here natural cosmetics as products whose efficacy is ascribed to their plant-derived ingredients."[59]

Natural skin products are products made with plant-based ingredients, including formulations of oils, butters, herbs, and essential oils. These ingredients have antioxidants, phytochemicals, and vitamins that benefit a person's skin. In addition, they promote moisturizing, soothing, and healing properties.

Natural skin care products generally cost more than commercial skin care products. The cost is because the farmers harvest the plants, which are then processed to make the ingredients. Then these ingredients are added and mixed with other plant ingredients to make the product. Machines are used; however, many steps in production are done by hand. These raw ingredients are from farms around the world, including farms from the continents of Africa and Asia.

Natural skin care products have shorter shelf lives than commercial products. One reason is due to the biodegradability of the ingredients. Natural ingredients will turn rancid quicker compared to synthetic ingredients.

Natural skin care products have evolved into different types and categories. Let's define the commonly used terms. Keep in mind that new terms are often developed.

a. Organic – Per the USDA, organic skin care products "need to contain at least 95 percent of formula in question must be organically produced, meaning those ingredients were grown without pesticides, artificial fertilizers, or any other synthetic ingredients."[60] If a product has the USDA organic labeling, that indicates that the food or other agricultural product has been produced according to the USDA organic standards.

b. Vegan – Vegan skin care products are also growing in popularity. Vegan skin products contain no animal ingredients or animal by-products. Presently, most of the products in natural skin care are vegan. Two examples of a non-vegan skin care ingredient are beeswax, a by-product of bees, and lard, used in some natural soap, made of pig fat.

c. Cruelty-free – Cruelty-free means the products are not tested on animals. There was a point when animal studies for human skin care products were the leading way to ensure the safety of the products. More recent research shows the "possibility that animal research is more costly and harmful, on the whole, than it is beneficial to human health."[61] Studies also show that the data collected from these animal studies are not as good of a predictor of the safety of humans as previously thought. Due to these findings, many natural skin care companies have taken a stance on not testing their products on animals.

d. Fair trade – Fair trade is another label you may see. Fair trade indicates that the product or ingredients from small farmers of international countries are purchased at a fair price. This agreement allows the countries involved to have a sustainable equal-trade relationship, which improves the lives of the farmers their communities.

e. Clean beauty – Clean beauty is a new term in the natural skin care industry. This term describes the use of "clean" ingredients that do not pose any threat or toxicity to human health. The difference between the terms "clean beauty" and "natural" and even "organic" is that "clean beauty products may contain synthetic or natural ingredients, all of which are tested and proven to be safe, and they don't contain toxins or any harmful ingredients."[62]

f. The FDA does not regulate the terminology "clean beauty." However, "the clean beauty industry avoids ingredients such as "chemical preservatives, parabens, sodium lauryl sulfate, glycol, phthalates, petrolatum, mineral oil, silicone, drying alcohol, fragrances and dyes."[63] Cosmeceuticals – Cosmeceuticals comprise another category of products in the cosmetic world. They are

> a cross between cosmetics and pharmaceuticals. Cosmeceuticals use biologically active ingredients to enhance the skin's beauty and health, particularly aging skin. You often find cosmeceuticals in medical spas, aesthetic offices, and some doctors' offices. Currently, the term cosmeceuticals is not defined by the FDA, therefore not fully regulated.

I am a preacher of natural skin care products; they are what I use on my skin and my family's skin. However, we must be mindful that not all natural products are safe or beneficial in certain situations. For example, a few citrus essential oils can cause photosensitivity. These essential oils are great for natural skin care products that wash off but not for skin care products meant to stay on the skin. Another example would be certain natural oils. Some are great for the body but can cause clogged pores if used on the face. Natural skin care makers follow formulas to ensure there is not an abundance of a natural ingredient that can cause irritation or harm if added at a high-enough percentage to a product.

Now, many natural skin care products use a preservative, mainly in water-based products or products that will come in contact with water, as they can be breeding grounds for bacteria, molds, and fungi. Also, these products have to compete with the shelf lives of the other products in the stores. They have to last there for at least six months to a year. Since the natural skin care movement, preservatives have evolved over the years to include preservatives that are not harmful and preservatives that are plant-based. Studies also show that many natural ingredients have innate anti-bacterial, antiviral, and antifungal properties; to what extent is still to be determined.

Many natural skin care creators stick to the absolutely no synthetic ingredients rule; however, this is not a rule for natural skin care makers. Some natural skin care products contain about 5–10 percent synthetic ingredients, such as fragrance oil and colorant. Many synthetic fragrance oils are safe for the skin, eyes, and lips, similar to skin-safe colorants. The attributes that attract people to skin products are scent, color, and feel. Many natural skin care makers stick to only essential oils or non-scented products; however, it is not unlikely for a natural product to have fragrance oils. To make sure the products you use are made of natural ingredients, read the ingredient list. Then, look up any unknown ingredients. Ingredients on products are labeled in order of percentage from highest to lowest. Finally, decide if you are okay with using a natural skin care product with essential oils, fragrance, colorants, or none of the above.

Chapter 3

The Natural Skin Care Movement

WHY NATURAL SKIN CARE: HEALTH

In recent years, there has been a great interest in natural skin care products. There are many different reasons for this movement. My motivation was health. While I was in medical school and residency, I started to make a transition to healthier products. I began to look at the list of ingredients for hair and skin care products. Many products had a list of fifteen-plus ingredients. As I researched the names of these ingredients, I learned that most had no health benefits. Some were even hazardous to my health. I became frustrated that I could not find products with fewer of these chemicals. I believe many others felt my frustration. These ingredients were not helping to moisturize, soothe, heal, or protect the skin. Also, many reports started discussing harmful chemicals in skin care products, including chemicals that can potentially cause endocrine and reproductive problems and cancer-associated risks.

Around the time I was making my transition, Chris Rock produced a documentary film called *Good Hair*. It documented him learning about the black woman's hair care regimen and experiences to answer his daughter's question, "Why don't I have good hair?" Her question was referring to why her hair was curly and not straight. In order to obtain a straight-hair look, black women often apply a chemical straightener. I remember watching this movie, happy I decided to stop chemically altering my hair but baffled at the health risks associated with using these products.

One study called "Hair Relaxer Use and Risk of Uterine Leiomyomata in African-American Women" shows a correlation between hair relaxers and uterine leiomyomata, which are commonly known as uterine fibroids. This study states that phthalates, which can be absorbed through the skin and inhaled, have estrogen effects in animal and cell models. Often, phthalates are added to the ingredient list as "fragrance." This chemical and other chemicals within the lye or no-lye hair relaxers can seep into the scalp by chemical burns caused by the product itself.[64]

More studies show that, in general, "women use more products than men, and products marketed towards women of color contain more hazardous materials than those marketed towards white women."[65] A further breakdown showed that African American women also spend more money on hair and skin products compared to women of other races. As a black woman, I grew up learning the importance of caring for my skin and my hair. Many black women know that healthy hair and skin require maintenance. Unfortunately, what was not well-known are the actual effects of some of the ingredients used to make many hair and skin care products marketed to black women. Now that this information is coming to the surface, many women are looking for alternatives and healthier options.

People with chronic conditions are also looking for healthier options. This search can be due to their belief that their skin care product was a risk factor contributing to their illness or worsening their disease. Either way, there are healthier options in skin care. With the news stating that ingredients in daily skin care products may have cancer-causing properties, a person with cancer or a family history of cancer will be looking for a more holistic option. People with autoimmune diseases may also look for a more holistic approach to managing their flare-ups.

WHY NATURAL SKIN CARE: ENTREPRENEURSHIP

Another cause for the natural skin care movement is entrepreneurism. People, particularly women, are tapping into their creativity and solving their skin and family's skin problems. Similar to the nineteenth century, women figure that if they have this problem, someone else in the country may have the same problem. As a result, many skin care companies started in a kitchen or a basement with a need to solve a skin care problem.

I started making skin care products in a small green kitchen. It was not the prettiest green—I remember it was more like a forest green. By this time, I was in my sports medicine fellowship training. As busy as I was that year, I am not sure how I managed to start brainstorming and creating products. It was definitely out of pure necessity; I became so passionate about the ingredients I put in my hair that it was not an option for me—I had to make the change. As I put on my research hat, I realized that I could probably make these products and use natural ingredients.

The first two products I created were my shea butter hair cream and hair oil. My hair oil became a hair and body oil, as it worked to moisturize my hair and body, leaving both soft, glowing, and healthy. I placed it in a large squirt bottle. With these two products, my hair was growing and healthy. After I started using my shea butter hair cream and hair and body oil regularly, I began looking closely at my skin products. I realized that the same harmful ingredients I was trying to avoid in my hair products were also in my skin products. So, I started to tweak my shea butter hair cream to make a body butter with the researched ingredients that would be benefit my skin. I followed this up by making a natural lip balm.

The summer after graduating from my yearlong sports medicine fellowship program was when I decided to make my transition out of my routine skin care into the products I was making. This transition included swapping out the store-bought lotion and lip balm for homemade body butter and lip balm. I continued to use my homemade shea butter cream and hair and body oil for my hair. I dabbled in natural shampoo and shampoo alternatives. I would go back and forth between purchasing "clean" shampoos and conditioners and using the ones I made at home.

My skin care products became a hit with my family and friends, as I often gift them products for birthdays and holidays. I started to hear the phrase "You should sell this!" a lot from my friends. Never before did I consider selling the products. It was not a thought in my mind. I was focusing on solving my problem. With a little push and great reviews from people who tried my products, I soon decided to start selling my creations. I had perfected my body butter and lip balm recipes by this time. However, I wanted to include an additional product, natural soap. So, I put my research hat back on and learned everything about making natural soap. I started to sway toward no-lye soap; however, I soon realized that the lye (an alkali) is needed to make natural soaps.

So, I set off to my garage, as I was no longer in the house with the green kitchen, to make soap.

Since my first product, I have made many skin care products, including scrubs, bath salts, bath bombs, and even shaving and beard products. Every natural skin care creator is different in their purpose. My purpose through the years is as solid as it was in the forest green kitchen. I make products out of necessity. We need to decrease chemicals and synthetic ingredients in our skin care and hair care products. I knew I could not keep these products I was making to myself. I had to share them with my family and friends, and now I share them with the world.

WHY NATURAL SKIN CARE: SUPPORT OF SMALL BUSINESSES

The natural skin care movement, I believe, was started by people who did not want to continue using the commercial skin care products stocked in the store aisles. These individuals knew there had to be better options. As a result, many of these individuals became creators and formulators of natural skin care products. People who support them appreciate the person behind the brand and their craftsmanship.

Before starting medical school, I never thought of myself as a business owner or an entrepreneur. I did not foresee owning a medical practice. I may have started making skin care products for my own personal needs; it also became my creative outlet from the stress of fellowship training. The idea of being an entrepreneur became more intriguing after completing my sports medicine fellowship and starting my first position as an attending physician. I may have been yearning to use the creative right side of my brain to balance the medical, analytical left side of my brain. Ultimately, I needed something that I had more control and creative power over and that served and helped people differently.

As we continue to move toward a more technological world with products easily bought with a smartphone swipe, I tend to want to learn how to make necessary daily products from scratch. It can be a lost art—the art of passing down recipes and ingredients through generations and generations. I also am reminded that the key elements used in many of these synthetic commercial products come from studying and synthesizing plant molecules. It all goes back to nature, where the medicinal aspect of medicine originated.

People started to learn about the conditions of animals in the testing laboratories and became concerned about product testing on animals. This concern led to the cruelty-free designation you now see on product labels and websites. Natural skin care products are safer and can be used without rigorous animal testing. All in all, people are concerned about how skin care products will affect their health, the health of animals, and the world in general.

THE MOVEMENT OF THE SKIN CARE MARKET

Many small business ventures have started with the natural skin care movement. New entrepreneurs who began making skin care products at home in their kitchens or basements to solve their and their families' skin care problems have turned to business ventures for people looking to serve others and sell their products. The global market has noticed, and you probably have seen that more natural ingredients are making their way into commercial skin care product labels and stores. Product branding also has changed as the focus shifts to cleaner beauty, organic products, fair trade, and non-animal cruelty products, as discussed before.

The market movement can also be because many stores are starting to restrict the sales of certain chemicals in the products they put on their shelves—stores mentioned before, such as Whole Foods, CVS, and Target. So now you are starting to see the word "natural" more often, as well as ingredients like shea butter, coconut oil, and avocado oil in the skin and health care products.

Large corporations are following the "natural" trend due to consumer requirements. In 2016, Procter and Gamble (P&G) published a list of 140 fragrance chemicals they would no longer use in their products. These chemicals, according to the Environmental Working Group (EWG), are linked to endocrine disruption, reproductive toxicity, and cancer.[66]

Chapter 4

How to Incorporate Natural Skin Care Products

ARE NATURAL INGREDIENTS THE NEW SKIN MEDICINE?

The skin consists of multiple defense and protection functions. First, the skin is a physical barrier to trauma, protecting the body from environmental conditions such as pollution and UV radiation. Second, the skin helps to keep out harmful microbes such as bacteria, fungi, and viruses. Third, the skin contains nerve roots that recognize sensation and pain. In addition, it helps regulate body temperature, maintain fluid balance, and assist certain endocrine functions.

With the skin functions, it makes sense that we should focus on maintaining our skin's daily health. Unfortunately, many do not know what it means to sustain healthy skin. Many women search for answers through social media, the internet, and non-healthcare expert blogs. As I did a few years back, many people are walking back and forth through the aisles of stores, trying to figure out how to obtain and maintain healthy skin.

The skin care products that we routinely place on our skin should have components promoting healthy skin. At a time, skin care products were "the medicinal preparations intended to be placed in contact with the various external parts of the human body that manifest beneficial topical actions and provide protection against degenerative skin conditions."[67] As a physician, I believe in the prevention of disease and the maintenance of good health. This concept should also apply to skin care. Routine skin care products should be designed to prevent, protect, cleanse, and heal the skin.

Protection: The sun's ultraviolet (UV) radiation causes increases in free radical formation. This free radical formation can lead to skin damage by decreasing skin elasticity and causing the wrinkling and leathery skin that is associated with early signs of aging. An unbalance of these free radical formations can also increase the risk of skin cancer. Skin cancer is in the top four most common cancers in the US as of 2022. The most common cause of skin cancer cases is exposure to UV rays from the sun. Prevention involves protecting the skin against damaging UV rays by decreasing excess exposure and using sunscreen. Prevention also includes stabilizing the free radical formation by using natural products containing antioxidants.

Protection and Cleansing: The skin is the first barrier to microbes such as bacteria, fungi, and viruses. It is essential to cleanse the skin to remove the harmful microbes; any dirty, excess skin oils; and debris. However, we do not want our cleansers to strip away all our natural moisture produced by the skin cells. Stripping away natural moisture is one cause of dry skin. This raises the question of whether you are using soap on your skin or detergent on your skin. It is best to use a natural soap that will cleanse the skin without stripping away all the moisture.

Moisturization: Moisturizing the skin is very important for skin health. A plant-based skin moisturizer should contain ingredients with antioxidants and vitamins that will support your skin cells with rebuilding nutrients. They may also contain ingredients that have antimicrobial properties. These act as an additional defense for the skin. Moisturizers also keep your skin soft and smooth; they decrease the skin drying by working as a protective layer on top of the skin that traps in moisture and is an added barrier to microbes. There are three types of moisturizers: humectants, occlusives, and emollients. A humectant will "attract water from two sources, from the dermis into the epidermis and in humid conditions from the environment."[68] Emollients are "mainly lipids and oils, which hydrate and improve the skin's softness, flexibility, and smoothness."[69] Occlusives are substances that physically block transdermal water loss in the outermost layer of the epidermis, called the *stratum corneum*.[70]

During the cold weather months, it is crucial to moisturize. These cold weather months can be especially rough on the skin. The cold outdoor air causes low humidity, which means very little water vapor is in the air. The low humidity draws out moisture from the outer layer of the skin, causing it to become dry. The dry skin can shrink the outer cell layer, causing rough skin that can even crack. The cracked skin can cause inflammation, making the skin feel itchy. Scratching this itchy skin can cause even more breaks within the skin, leading to infection pathways. This cascade effect is why it is crucial to maintain healthy skin during the winter months.

Healing: Healing the skin is one component not often discussed in the holistic sense. Can or do natural skin care products heal the skin? As a physician, I treat skin conditions with proven effective medications, especially for conditions that have worsened and need medication to resolve and maintain the condition. In addition, for skin conditions that are autoimmune-caused, applying just a topical plant-based product to it will not reach the root cause of the problem. That said, we should not overlook the properties of these natural plant-based ingredients. Many of these properties are used to make the prescription skin medications we use today. Also, the fact that these plant molecules are studied proves that beneficial properties are present.

We are discussing skin health from the outside. We also need to discuss skin health from the inside out. What we consume will affect our skin's health. As part of the skin care routine, water is an essential component of cell health. Water hydrates our body's cells, including the cells of our skin. Keeping the skin hydrated will maintain its elasticity, which helps to decrease the onset of dry and cracked skin. Foods such as vegetables and fruits are high in antioxidants, vitamins, omega fatty acids, and nutrients. These properties will not only benefit your overall health; they will also help the skin cells fight off free radical formations.

In the medical field, I do not believe it should be one or the other in terms of healing the skin with prescription medication or natural plant-based products. Instead, it should be a balance of both. However, the best way to maintain your skin health and decrease the need for prescription medication is to use trusted plant-based skin care products in your daily skin care routine.

Natural skin care companies focus on providing products with quality ingredients. There are staple ingredients in natural skin care products, including natural butter, carrier oils, waxes, herbs, and essential oils. These ingredients are what you should look for when purchasing products:

Natural butters – These are butters that come from tree nuts. The nut contains properties including antioxidant, moisturizing, and healing properties. That nut is then turned into a solid form and used to make butters.

Common plant-based butters: shea butter, cocoa butter, mango butter, and kokum butter

Carrier oils – Carrier oils are oils made from nuts and fruits. They are pressed to make an oil that contains skin-benefiting properties such as antioxidants and vitamins. These oils also have moisturizing properties. In some countries, oils are also known for their medicinal properties. Natural plant-based oils add a protective barrier to the skin and provide an occlusive effect, allowing the skin to retain moisture.

Common plant-based carrier oils: almond oil, jojoba oil, soybean oil, avocado oil, coconut oil, olive oil, castor oil, grape seed oil, rose hip oil, babassu oil, and argan oil

Essential oils – Essential oils have been around for centuries and are known for their many beneficial and healing properties. They are used in aromatherapy, diffusers, and skin care products.

Some of the most common essential oils for the skin: lavender, chamomile, sandalwood, rosemary, geranium, frankincense, tea tree, lemongrass, peppermint, eucalyptus, patchouli, carrot seed, and ylang essential oils

Herbs – Herbs have also been used in skin care for centuries due to their individual healing properties.

Common herbs used in skin care: lavender buds, chamomile flower, calendula flower, peppermint leaf, and rosemary leaf

Clays – Clays also provide healing properties and are great for removing dead skin cells. Clays absorb impurities from the pores. This absorption can help control acne by balancing the oil production of the skin. Natural clays also boost the skin's elasticity and collagen production. Be mindful of unnatural clays with colorant, which does not have a beneficial purpose for the skin.

Common natural clays in skin care: rhassoul clay, bentonite clay, French green clay, and kaolin clay

Exfoliants – Exfoliating is the process of removing dead cells from the skin. Excess dead skin cells can clog the pores and cause rough skin when not removed.

Common exfoliants used in natural skin care: sugar, salt, herbs, seeds, and colloidal oatmeal

There have been claims made that natural plant-based ingredients are not well-studied compared to synthetic skin care ingredients. However, there are studies on natural ingredients proving their beneficial skin properties. Through research, I found studies performed on the properties of plants that benefit the skin's health. Below, I provide a breakdown on the ingredients, their beneficial properties, and some of the researched conducted.

Olive oil – Olive oil is extracted from the fruits of the olive tree, *Olea europaea*, either by mechanical or chemical processes. It has been used for hair and skin care in many cultures for centuries. This popularity is due to the abundance of antioxidant properties it contains. Olive oil "consists mainly of oleic acid, with smaller quantities of other fatty acids such as linoleic acid and palmitic acid. More than two hundred different chemical compounds have been detected in olive oil, including sterols, carotenoids, triterpenic alcohols, and phenolic compounds."[71]

The most abundant antioxidants in olive oil are hydrophilic phenols; "the phenolic contents have antioxidant properties higher than those of vitamin E." Olive oil is the most commonly used plant-based oil in hair and skin care. It is also the most routinely used oil in the diet of many people.[72]

In hair and skin care, olive oil can be used on its own for moisturizing and hydrating the hair and moisturizing the skin. One of the earliest forms of using olive oil in skin care was using it as the main ingredient in natural soap. Dating back to the eleventh century and possibly earlier was the first form of olive oil-based soap. The most popularly known olive oil-based soap is the Castile soap, named after the Castile region in Spain.

Olive oil can be used in many ways on the skin and hair. It is a versatile oil that can be added to all natural skin care products. Olive oil can be used as a solo oil for your hair and skin; however, I prefer mixing it with other oils, as it can be used for hair moisturizer or deep conditioning and in body butters, body lotions, and exfoliating scrubs.

Coconut oil – Coconut oil is extracted from the kernel or meat of mature harvested from the coconut palm, *Cocos nucifera*. Coconut oil is high in fatty acids, such as "lauric acid (49 percent), myristic acid (18 percent), palmitic acid (8 percent), caprylic acid (8 percent), capric acid (7 percent), oleic acid (6 percent), linoleic acid (2 percent), and stearic acid (2 percent)."[73]

Studies have shown the benefits of coconut oils on the skin. For example, in one study on "pediatric patients with mild to moderate Atopic dermatitis, topical applications of virgin coconut oil show effectiveness in decreasing the severity of the disease and improving barrier function."[74] Improving the barrier function of the skin helps to decrease the amount of water loss, reduce the number of external irritants entering the deeper layers of the skin, and increase moisture retention.

Coconut oil applied topically was shown to promote wound healing by helping to increase new collagen formation. Collagen is a protein found in the skin cells that makes the skin strong and resilient while decreasing skin sagging and wrinkle formation. Collagen is also found in the body's bones, muscles, ligaments, and tendons. The repairing properties of coconut oil and its ability to help protect the skin from UV radiation make coconut oil an excellent choice of topical moisturizer for aging skin.

Studies also show the antimicrobial activities of coconut oil. Coconut oil contains a molecule called monolaurin that exhibits antiviral and antifungal activities. This molecule can potentially help prevent microbials from breaking through the skin barrier. I believe more studies are needed to explore these properties further. Nonetheless, coconut oil has shown itself to be a versatile oil for all age groups, protecting the skin's barrier, increasing moisture retention, increasing collagen production, and helping to prevent microbials from breaking through the outer skin cell layer.

Coconut oil is an oil that can be applied directly to the skin. Due to its abundant beneficial properties, it does not have to be mixed with additional plant-based oils or butters. It can be applied to the hair as a conditioner and directly on the skin as a moisturizer. It is a light oil that is solid at room temperature but melts quickly when applied to the skin. Coconut oil can also be mixed with other butters to form a multi-butter moisturizer. You will see coconut oil in many natural products, such as hair conditioners, body butters, body lotions, and lip balms.

Argan oil – Argan oil originates from Morocco. Argan oil comes from the argan tree, *Argania spinosa L.* The argan tree produces fruits. Within these fruits is the nut that holds the kernel. The kernel is extracted from the nut, then pressed to make the oil. The composition of Argan oil consists of "mono-unsaturated (80 percent) and saturated (20 percent) fatty acids, as well as polyphenols, tocopherols, sterols, squalene, and triterpene alcohols."[75]

Traditionally, argan oil has been utilized in the treatment of skin infections and in skin and hair care products. Daily topical application of argan oil has also been shown to improve skin elasticity and skin hydration by restoring the barrier function and maintaining the water-holding capacity.[76] This makes argan oil a great oil to use on aging skin. One property of the skin that diminishes as we age is the skin's elasticity.

As we age, our skin loses collagen and elastin. These two proteins are the building structures providing the skin with firmness and elasticity. Elastin helps your skin to stretch and bounce back. This makes argan oil an excellent plant-based oil for the face as well as the body. Argan oil is a light oil that can be used as a solo oil, especially on the face. However, it can be mixed with additional oils and butters for application on the skin and hair.

Avocado oil – Avocado oil, derived from the avocado tree, *Persea amehoiuiopricana,* is one of the few edible oils not derived from seeds. Instead, the oil is extracted from the pulp surrounding the seed. Avocado oil is composed of "linoleic acid (6.1–22.9 percent), linolenic acid (0.4–4.0 percent), and oleic acid (31.8–69.6 percent)."[77] It is also high in β-sitosterol, β-carotene, lecithin, minerals, and vitamins A, C, D, and E.[78]

Avocado oil is a plant-based oil that is "rapidly absorbed by the skin and has sunscreen properties."[79] Its antioxidant properties make it "an excellent source of enrichment for dry, damaged, or chapped skin."[80] Due to its penetrating effect on the skin, avocado oil is used in many massage oils, creams, and muscle oils. Avocado oil is also one of the most common oils used in natural soap making due to its ability to aid in providing a smoother, creamier lather.

Jojoba oil – Jojoba oil is derived from a long-lived, drought resistant, perennial plant. Jojoba oil is extracted from the seed of the fruit from the shrub *Simmondsia chinensis*. This plant grows in the southwestern United States and northwestern Mexico. Unlike other plant oils, jojoba oil has wax properties due to its mixtures of long chain esters, fatty acids, and fatty alcohols. Although jojoba is referred to as an oil, it is actually a liquid wax.

Jojoba oil is a humectant; it draws in moisture and seals in it by creating a protective layer over the skin. Due to its properties of broad-spectrum fatty acids such as oleic acid, linoleic acid, and arachidonic acid and its triglycerides, jojoba oil has good compatibility with the natural sebum in the human skin.[81]

Jojoba oil has beneficial properties, including "analgesic, antipyretic, anti-inflammatory, antioxidant, anti-bacterial and anti-parasitic properties."[82] Due to its high makeup of wax esters, jojoba oil is an excellent option for repairing altered skin barriers, as seen in seborrheic dermatitis, eczematous dermatitis, atopic dermatitis, and acne.[83] Its ability to absorb well into the skin makes jojoba oil a versatile oil for moisturizers and sunscreens. Also, its anti-inflammatory properties positively affect "skin conditions including skin infection, skin aging, and wound healing."[84]

Jojoba oil's properties are so similar to the skin's sebum. As a result, it absorbs fully, leaving no oily residue. With this said, jojoba oil can be applied directly to the face and used in massage oils, lip balms, and body moisturizer mixtures.

Almond oil – Almond oil is extracted from the seed of the almond tree, *Oleum amygdalae.* Almond oil has emollient and moisturizing properties. Emollients have properties that soften and soothe the skin. Almond oil is used on all skin types to improve complexion and skin tone. Its use has been present for centuries in "ancient Chinese, Ayurvedic and Greco-Persian schools of medicine to treat dry skin conditions such as psoriasis and eczema."[85]

Almond oil can be used alone to moisturize the face. It can also be combined with other oils and plant-based butters in lotions, body butters, scrubs, and lip balms. It also pairs well in massage oils because of its light texture and how well it absorbs into the skin.

Rose hip oil – Rose hip oil is extracted from the seeds of the fruit from the rose hip bush, *Rosa canina L.* Rose hip oil is high in unsaturated fatty acids, such as "linoleic acid (35.9–54.8 percent), followed by α-linolenic acid (16.6–26.5 percent), and oleic acid (14.7–22.1 percent)."[86] It contains antioxidants such as tocopherols and carotenoids. With the combination of fatty acids and antioxidants, rose hip oil is an excellent anti-inflammatory and antioxidant ingredient.

Rose hip oil is commonly used as a facial oil for antiaging the skin. It is used alone or in combination with other plant-based oils. There are two main types of aging skin—one is the skin alteration associated with the normal aging process, and the other is the skin alteration related to excessive UV radiation from sun exposure.

German chamomile oil – German chamomile oil is extracted from the flower of the chamomile plant, *Matricaria recutita.* Chamomile is high in antioxidants such as flavonoids. Flavonoids are considered phytonutrients found in plants. In addition, they contain anti-inflammatory and antioxidative properties, which contribute to the medicinal properties of chamomile.

Traditionally, chamomile has been used for centuries as an anti-inflammatory, an antioxidant, a mild astringent, and healing medicine. As a traditional medicine in skin care, it treats wounds, ulcers, eczema, skin irritation, bruises, burns, diaper rash, and cracked nipples, to name a few. Chamomile is also widely used to treat inflammations of the skin and mucous membranes and for various bacterial infections of the skin, oral cavity, gums, and respiratory tract.

Studies on chamomile and its effects on the treatment of atopic eczema show topical applications of chamomile to be "moderately effective in the treatment of atopic eczema. It was about 60 percent as effective as 0.25 percent hydrocortisone cream. Roman chamomile of the Manzana type (Kamillosan (R)) may ease discomfort associated with eczema when applied as a cream containing chamomile extract."[87]

Chamomile has positive effects on wound healing, which has been shown in some human studies. In one double-blind trial on fourteen patients who underwent dermabrasion for their tattoos, chamomile was shown to be statistically effective in encouraging wound drying and speeding the epithelialization of the skin.[88]

There are different ways to use chamomile in skin care. Chamomile can be used in extract and oil forms. Chamomile's properties are extracted "from the dry flowers of chamomile by using water, ethanol or methanol as solvents and corresponding extracts are known as aqueous, ethanolic (alcoholic) and/or methanolic extracts."[89] Chamomile extract is added to skin care products such as lotions, body butters, salves, and body oils. Chamomile can be used as an herb in an herbal oil infusion. An herbal oil infusion incorporates a healing herb of choice into an oil. The oil will absorb the healing properties of the herb either by incubating for six to eight weeks or by *double* boiler heating method. This oil can be applied to the skin, made into a salve, or added to products.

Shea butter – Shea butter is extracted from the kernels of the shea tree, *Vitellaria paradoxa*. The kernels are pounded, ground into an oily chocolate paste, and then boiled. This process helps to remove impurities, leaving the oil that is shea butter. Shea butter contains "triglycerides with oleic, stearic, linoleic, and palmitic fatty acids, as well as unsaponifiable compounds."[90] This butter is often used in hair and skin care "due to its high percentage of triterpenes, tocopherol, phenols, and sterols, which possesses potent anti-inflammatory and antioxidant properties."[91]

Shea butter is an emollient and a moisturizer. Studies show that shea butter helps repair dry, inflamed skin caused by dermatitis.[92] Shea butter can be an emollient for skin conditions such as eczema. For example, in a study comparing shea butter to Vaseline on how well each clears up eczema using a scale from zero to five, "shea butter took a three down to a one, while Vaseline only took a three down to a two."[93] Further studies on atopic dermatitis show that creams "containing shea butter extract had the same efficacy as ceramide-precursor product."[94] Ceramides are lipids (fats) produced by the skin. They help hold the skin cells together. In youthful skin, ceramide is at high concentrations. However, as the skin ages, the amount of ceramide production decreases, which, along with the skin damage caused by UV radiation from the sun, leads to dry, damaged, and wrinkled skin.

Shea butter is a versatile butter that is solid at room temperature and melts when you apply it to the skin. Shea butter can be used alone on the skin or combined with additional plant-based butters and oils to produce lotions, body butters, soaps, and lip balms. Shea butter was the first plant-based butter I experimented with when starting to make skin care products, and today it remains one of the staple ingredients of Nature's Purée products.

Sunflower seed oil – Sunflower seed oil, derived from the sunflower plant, *Helianthus annus*, is extracted from the sunflower seed by grinding the seed, pressing it, and drawing out the oil. Sunflower oil primarily consists of oleic and linoleic acids. These fatty acid concentrations are higher in sunflower oil as compared to olive oil. Sunflower oil is an excellent option for hair and skin care products. Sunflower seed oil improves the skin's hydration by preserving the integrity of the *stratum corneum*, which is the outermost layer of the skin. In particular, linoleic acid enhances keratinocyte proliferation and lipid synthesis, strengthening the skin barrier's repair system.[95] Keratinocytes are the dominant cells that are found in the skin's epidermis. Keratinocytes help the skin repair process by migrating, proliferating, and differentiating into cells that restore the skin barrier.

Natural oils such as sunflower, sesame, and safflower seed oil have been suggested as good options for their use in promoting skin barrier homeostasis. In a pilot study conducted of neonatal skin topically treated with sunflower seed oil or olive oil, there were no differences in lipid structure changes, transepidermal water loss, hydration, skin surface pH, erythema, or skin assessment scores between the olive oil and sunflower oil groups.[96]

Sunflower seed oil is high in antioxidants such as vitamin E and beta-carotene. It also contains vitamin A, vitamin C, vitamin K, and vitamin D. Human trial studies show good evidence of the benefits of sunflower seed oil, such as: "antifungal treatment in adults' onychomycosis, infection preventing in premature neonates, atopic dermatitis treatment in infants and babies, 'dry skin' and 'scaly skin' treatment in adults and elders with EFA deficiencies, anti-wrinkling and antiaging properties, improving gingival condition, and psoriasis complementary treatment."[97] Sunflower seed oil can be used directly on the skin, including the face, or mixed with additional plant-based oils and butters. It also makes for a great addition to ointments and salves for sensitive skin, especially for children and the elderly.

Grape seed oil – Grape seed oil is extracted from the seeds of grapes, *Vitis vinifera*, either by cold-pressed processes or the use of a chemical solvent. Grape seed oil contains properties high in antioxidants such as phenolic compounds, resveratrol, and vitamin E.

Many animal studies on grape seed oil have shown it to aid in wound healing. In particular, the plant compound resveratrol, an antioxidant, has shown "faster wound contraction, enhanced synthesis of vascular endothelial growth factor, and greater connective tissue deposition."[98] Resveratrol contains antimicrobial activities against bacteria such as "*Staphylococcal aureus*, *Enterococcus faecalis*, and *Pseudomonas aeruginosa* in the animal model studies."[99] On human skin, resveratrol applied topically is said to increase cathelicidin production. This production induces antimicrobial peptides and "inhibits the growth of *Staphylococcal aureus*." More studies are being conducted to isolate resveratrol from grape seed oil.[100]

Grape seed oil is an oil that can be used solo the face, since it is a lightweight oil, it does not clog the pores. It can be applied after a cleanser as a single oil or mixed with additional plant- based oils and butters.

Safflower seed oil – Safflower seed oil is expeller-pressed from safflower seeds, which are derived from the safflower plant, *Carthamus tinctorius*. Safflower seed oil contains a large amount of fatty acids, such as polyunsaturated linoleic acid and monounsaturated oleic acid.[101]

Safflower seed oil has analgesic and antipyretic effects, which can help reduce pain and fever. This is due to its anti-inflammatory properties.[102]

Soybean oil – Soybean oil is extracted for the soybean, *Glycine max*, by a chemical solvent. It contains phytosterols, anthocyanin, antioxidants such as vitamin E, and omega fatty acids. Soybean oil can work as a sealant that seals in the moisture, keeping the skin hydrated and soft. Soybean is often combined with additional plant-based oils and butters.

Soybean oil extract has positive effects on the human skin barrier. For example, soybean oil extract topically decreases transepidermal water loss of the skin's forearm.[103] This is due to its properties, such as soy phytosterol. In addition, soybean, particularly black soybean, has anti-inflammatory and antioxidant properties. These properties are most likely due to its anthocyanins, which help give the black soybean its color.

Peanut oil – Peanut oil is extracted from the peanut plant, *Arachis hypogaea*, using cold-press methods or chemical solvents. The beneficial components of peanut oil consist of linolenic acid, stearic acid, and oleic acid. Peanut oil is rich in antioxidants such as vitamin E. This property makes peanut oil an emollient, helping to soothe and soften dry skin.

Topical skin use of peanut oil can "have hydrating effects in human skin without significantly increasing transepidermal water loss."[104] It can also help protect the skin from the harmful effects of UV radiation. As peanut oil gains attention, the question becomes: how safe is topical peanut oil on the skin of a person who has a peanut allergy or sensitivity? Some studies have suggested that "refined peanut oil-containing preparation is safe for topical use, even in persons who are sensitive to peanuts."[105] With that said, and with many other oils to choose from, I would recommend a different plant-based oil if one is allergic or sensitive to peanuts.[106]

Sesame oil – Sesame oil comes from the sesame plant, *Sesamum indicum*. It is extracted through cold-pressing by crushing the seeds at low temperatures to release the oils. Sesame seeds contain polyphenols called lignans. These lignans, such as sesamin, sesamolin, and sesaminol, exhibit antioxidative activity.[107]

In traditional Taiwanese medicine, sesame oil has been used to relieve inflammatory pain in joints and wounds.[108] Studies on limb trauma show that applying sesame oil on the skin can help "lower the severity of pain and reduce the frequency of nonsteroidal anti-inflammatory drug use in patients with limb trauma."[109] Topical sesame oil also protects the skin from UV radiation."[110]

Borage oil – Borage oil is expressed from the seeds of the borage plant, *Borago officinalis*. Borage oil is high in essential fatty acids, which help to improve the skin's structure and function. Specifically, the linoleic acid found in borage oil "contributes to its therapeutic actions in atopic dermatitis."[111] In research studies, "topical application of borage oil in infants and children with seborrheic dermatitis or atopic dermatitis has been shown to normalize skin barrier function."[112]

Borage oil is best used in combination with a carrier plant-based oil such as almond oil, avocado oil, or olive oil. It can also be added to lotions and moisturizers. It is one oil that has shown positive outcomes in the treatment of seborrheic dermatitis and atopic dermatitis in infants and children. It will also have similar beneficial effects on aging skin.

Oat oil – Oat oil is extracted from the kernels of *Avena sativa* in a process called ethanolic extraction. This process allows the oils to be extracted while maintaining their beneficial properties. Oat oil "consists of 36–46 percent linoleic and 28–40 percent oleic acid," which aid in the repair and protection of the skin barrier.[113] For centuries, colloidal oat was used as a topical treatment for skin conditions such as "skin rashes, erythema, burns, itch, and eczema."[114] In addition, colloidal oat extracts exhibit direct antioxidant and anti-inflammatory activities, which "may explain the efficacy of lotions containing colloidal oatmeal."[115] Oats contain avan-thramides, an antioxidant molecule with anti-inflammatory, antiproliferative, and anti-itching activities. These properties make oat oil an excellent oil for moisturizing and nourishing the skin.[116]

Pomegranate seed oil – Pomegranate seed oil comes from the seed of the pomegranate fruit, *Punica granatum.* It is extracted using the cold-pressed method. Pomegranate seed oil contains fatty acids such as linoleic acid and oleic acid. It also includes "phenolic compounds, phytosterols, and lipid-soluble fractions."[117] Pomegranate seed oil contains antioxidant and anti-inflammatory properties. It has positive effects on wound healing, aging skin and skin cancer in animal model studies.[118]

Pomegranate seed oil is highly antioxidant and anti-inflammatory, making it a perfect oil for the face, as it helps to increase the face's elasticity, which helps decrease the signs of aging. In addition, pomegranate seed oil is added with additional oils to produce moisturizers, lotions, lip balms, and facial serums.

Bitter apricot oil – Bitter apricot oil comes from the apricot kernel from the apricot plant, *Semen Armeniacae amarum.* The oil is made by either the cold-pressed or the solvent extraction method. Apricot kernels are composed of mainly fatty acids such as oleic acid. They are also high in "proteins, fibers, phenolic compounds, vitamins, and minerals."[119] These known properties give apricot kernels "antioxidant, antibacterial and antiparasitic effects."[120]

Bitter apricot seed is known in Eastern medicine as a treatment for skin conditions. It has the ability to rid the skin of damaged cells in a process called apoptosis. Apoptosis in the human skin removes old and damaged cells such as keratinocytes. Keratinocytes are the cells located in the epidermis skin layer that produce keratin. Keratin is a structural protein found in hair, skin, and nails. Apricot oil may have the potential to treat psoriasis "given its pro-apoptotic effect on human keratinocytes."[121] Apricot oil is a versatile oil that can be used on the whole body solo or combined with other plant-based oils.

Calendula oil – Calendula oil is derived from a plant also known as pot marigold, *Calendula officinalis*. Calendula oil is made through natural oil extraction by infusing the flowers in a carrier oil. Calendula is abundant in beneficial compounds such as terpenoids, terpenes, carotenoids, flavonoids, and polyunsaturated fatty acids.[122]

The calendula plant is known for its wound-healing potential. It is one of the "remedies for burns (including sunburns), abrasions, bruises, and cutaneous inflammatory diseases."[123] Studies performed on topical "preparations containing seven different types of marigold and rosemary extracts revealed that such creams are effective in experimentally induced irritant contact dermatitis when tested on healthy human volunteers."[124]

Calendula-infused herbal oil makes salves, ointments, and lip balms. The herbal oil mix is added to moisturizers, lotions, and soaps. In addition, due to the soothing and healing properties of calendula, you can often find it in baby products, breastfeeding salves, and ointments.

Aloe vera – Aloe vera, *Barbados aloe*, is a succulent plant known as a "wonder plant." The aloe vera gel is extracted by cutting away the spiky sides and skin. Aloe vera is abundant in beneficial properties, containing seventy-five active compounds. These compounds include "vitamins, enzymes, minerals, sugars, lignin, saponins, salicylic acids, and amino acids."[125] Aloe vera contains vitamins A, C, and E, which are potent antioxidants. In addition, it has anti-inflammatory properties through its multiple enzyme pathways. It also has antibacterial and antiseptic properties through compounds such as salicylic acid and saponins.

Aloe vera has healing properties that increase the collagen synthesis of the skin after topical use. This collagen synthesis helps to accelerate wound contraction and increase the strength of the scar tissue. Aloe vera also protects against sun damage. It is the most common natural topical product used for minor sunburns. Aloe vera is an excellent moisturizer that has antiaging effects. The long chain of sugar molecules such as *m*ucopolysaccharides in aloe vera "help in binding moisture into the skin."[126] This plant can "stimulate fibroblast, which produces the collagen and elastin fibers, making the skin more elastic and less wrinkled."[127] It can improve dry skin by making the epidermis cells sticky, leading to softer skin. The additional properties of aloe vera, such as its amino acids and zinc, can soften rough skin and tighten the skin pores, respectively.[128] Aloe vera gel can be applied directly to the skin, especially for cases of sunburn, burns, and skin scars. The gel can also be applied to lotions, soaps, and body butter.

Natural ingredients aren't without side effects. When selecting a product, look first at the product ingredients. Are you allergic to any of the ingredients? If you are prone to skin reactions or are not sure how you would react to the product, do a spot test first. A spot test is when you apply a small amount of the product, usually on the arm, to see if there is a reaction. Reactions can range from itchiness to rashes or redness of the skin.

Look for any product disclaimers. A product disclaimer is a "statement used by sellers, marketers, and manufacturers to let consumers know what to expect from their products or product reviews."[129] Natural skin care products are not substitutions for skin conditions needing specific medical attention and treatments. For example, if you have an abscess or cellulitis of the skin, this condition can worsen very quickly and lead to a systemic infection called sepsis. Also, some skin conditions are manifestations of an underlying illness, such as the bulls-eye rash (erythema migrans) seen with Lyme disease. If you develop a skin rash or infection, it is best to consult with your doctor first.

Some ingredients are not safe during pregnancy or breastfeeding. For example, some essential oils help to combat morning sickness and nausea and promote relaxation and a good night's sleep.[130] However, some essential oils can cause uterine contractions, resulting in miscarriage or preterm labor. To be safe, avoid essential oils that can pose possible harm during pregnancy and breastfeeding.

THE NATURAL SKIN CARE ROUTINE

When we think about our health, we should also consider our skin's health. As a physician, I regularly recommend maintaining good health by eating nutritious foods and exercising. However, maintaining healthy skin also is a part of maintaining good overall health. A skin care routine is a sequence of actions that are done regularly, not only on certain occasions. A skin routine will help to maintain and seal in moisture, soothe and soften the skin, provide the skin with the nutrients and antioxidants it needs, and decrease breakouts of chronic skin conditions. Here are my five components of a healthy skin care routine:

Natural Soap

Many soaps sold in the stores are synthetic detergents and not true soaps. These commercial soaps are harsh on the skin and can strip away the skin's natural moisturizer, making the skin feel and look dry. Natural soaps do not contain synthetic detergent; they are milder cleansers than commercial soaps and do not remove moisture from your skin. Natural soaps contain oils that help replenish lost moisture and provide your skin with vitamins and antioxidants helpful in cell repair.

Natural soap will cleanse your skin without stripping away all of your skin's moisture. Since it is made with oil, it will help replenish the skin with oils that contain vitamins and antioxidants beneficial to the skin. Some may think of natural soap as a luxury item that should be used on occasion. However, natural soaps should be used with each bath to maximize its benefits and maintain healthy skin.

Ingredients in natural soap comprise a mixture of plant-based butters and oils. Natural soaps can also contain exfoliants, clays, and plant products such as aloe, sea moss, and avocado, to name a few–all of which will have an additive benefit to the skin.

Natural Moisturizer

A natural moisturizer such as body butter, cream, or lotion contains a combination of natural butters and oils. These butters and oils are known as emollients. Emollients work as a barrier on the skin's surface; it helps to prevent dry skin by trapping in the moisture. These moisturizing butters and oils are also soothing to sensitive skin and contain antioxidants and vitamins that help in cell repair and diminish the appearance of aged skin.

Commonly used emollient butters are shea butter, cocoa butter, and coconut oil. Natural oils including olive oil, avocado oil, castor oil, almond oil, and jojoba oil are also excellent emollients. When choosing a moisturizer, I recommend checking the product labels to ensure that plant-based butters and oils make up the entire, or at least the majority, of the ingredients.

For best results, moisturize your skin twice daily in the morning and evening with natural body butter, cream, or lotion. This process will help protect your skin from losing water, help with cell repair, and soothe any sensitive skin.

Natural Exfoliator

Exfoliants are used to remove the top layer of dead cells from the skin. The cells of the body are constantly replenishing themselves. Many times, dead skin cells can lay on top of the new skin cells, clogging the pores and causing dry, dull, rough skin patches. Exfoliating will help to remove the excess dead cells, leaving your skin feeling and looking soft and smooth. It will also increase the effectiveness of natural moisturizers.

Exfoliants such as colloidal oatmeal, finely ground sugar, and finely ground sea salt are excellent exfoliants for dry and sensitive skin. Exfoliate the skin once per week or twice per month. Exfoliate your skin after rinsing off the soap from your body. Apply the exfoliate to your hand, massage it onto your body, and then rinse. After rinsing and padding dry with a towel, apply your skin moisturizer.

Natural Salve

A salve is a healing ointment. It is used for moisturizing dry skin, soothing burns such as sunburns and diaper rash, healing wounds and scars, and relieving musculoskeletal pain. Salves have two main ingredients. The first is an herb-infused oil. An herbal oil infusion is when a healing herb of choice is added to natural oil. The oil will absorb the herb's healing properties. The second is beeswax, or a plant-based wax. These waxes are emollients and humectants; they draw moisture into the skin and provide a protective layer that seals in the moisture. The herb-infused oil and wax are melted, mixed, and cooled to form the salve.

Salves with calendula and chamomile herb-infused oils are excellent for dry, sensitive skin due to their healing and soothing properties. Salves are most often used in trouble areas such as the hands, feet, elbows, and knees. These areas tend to be drier and coarser than other body areas. Apply herb-infused salve, as needed, to these areas or at least twice a day to help heal, soothe, and moisturize.

Natural Lip Balm

We cannot forget the lips, as this area of the body can become very dry and chapped, causing cuts and pain. Natural lip balms containing butters such as shea butter and cocoa butter and oils such as olive oil and avocado oil can help soothe dry lips, providing them with moisture throughout the day. This moisture is sealed with a humectant such as beeswax or plant-based wax. The best time during the day to apply lip balm is in the morning and before bed to help keep the lips soft, smooth, and moisturized.

HOW TO TRANSITION TO NATURAL SKIN CARE PRODUCTS

This book may have convinced you to transition some or all of your skin care products to natural plant-based products. If so, let's talk about how to make the transition. I decided to transition gradually away from commercial skin care products. Going cold turkey is another option. Since my natural skin care journey started with my hair, those products were the first to be transitioned. I started with my first creations, hair butter and a hair and body oil, which became my two staple hair products. Then I changed my shampoo and conditioner to all-natural and some others with non-harmful synthetic ingredients.

Once comfortable and happy with my hair products, I tweaked my hair butter to make a body butter. I started to use my body butter alongside the store-bought lotion. When I felt ready, I stopped purchasing the lotion. Instead, I just walked past what used to be an irresistible aisle for me in the supermarket. This transition was smooth; I quickly adapted to using only my products and was happy with the results.

The next transition was my lip balm. I replaced all my store-bought lip balms with Nature's Purée balms. This transition was the easiest, as I was empowered by the transformations I had already undertaken. I usually carry a lip balm in several frequently used bags. I did an even swap and never looked back.

I started making natural soap about one to two years after my transition. However, before then, I changed my body soap to one with minimum synthetic ingredients. One of my most challenging transitions—which, to be honest, I still struggle with to this day—was natural deodorant. Unfortunately, I have not found one that works to my liking. Maybe Nature's Purée will create a natural deodorant; till then, the search is still on.

I recommend a gradual approach to transitioning your skin care products. First, find a skin care company you like. This will require trying different products and different companies. You will want to have a go-to product and/or company that you can rely on. There is always room for trying different products and pampering yourself with luxurious natural products; however, some of these products can have a higher price point due to the ingredients used. This is why I recommend finding a go-to product that is affordable for you, easily assessable via e-commerce or a store, and able to give you the same results with each use. Once you find the products you like, start to decrease the use of the products you wish to transition out of using. Then stop purchasing those products. Remember that you must maintain the routine of applying the products for healthy skin. It is the consistency that will show you the greatest results.

I started a skin care company because my family and friends saw the same results on their skin as I saw on my skin. That was when I realized I had products that could help people, and I had to share them with everyone. At that time, I had just started my family of now three children. Using Nature's Purée products on their skin has been a blessing, as I am confident in knowing that I am not using potentially harmful ingredients on their skin.

When you start making small changes to your health, even if you start with skin care products, you can continue to make changes from the outside and inside. You will become more invested in keeping your body healthy. Not only will you pay attention to what you are putting on your body, but you'll also be noticing what you are putting in your body and how you are caring for your body by becoming more physically active. You will become more attuned to nature, finding ways out of your busy day to enjoy nature, even if it is a ten-minute walk.

After transitioning to natural skin products, I became more aware of additional harmful ingredients in foods and cleaning products. I was always health-conscious; however, I was on the road to all-around wellness before I knew it.

I hope for you, as this book concludes, to have gained more inside into skin care's past, present, and future. The future is promising, as I believe there will continue to be an increase in the regulation of harmful ingredients in skin care, and natural skin care products will be widely accepted as the norm. Skin health is part of your overall health, and what we need to help maintain our overall health comes from nature.

If you are interested in learning more about natural skin care or starting a new skin care routine, visit us at www.naturespuree.com. Follow us on all the major social medial platforms @naturespuree. If you have a question, feel free to email at orders@naturespuree.com.

WHAT ARE THE CUSTOMERS SAYING ABOUT NATURE'S PURÉE?

Forever customer

Review by Tai R. on 2 Jan 2022 review stating Forever customer

I have been a loyal supporter of Nature's Purée for over six years. The products are handmade and all-natural. This family-owned small business is one of my absolute favorites ever. I will continue to trust my skin care to this brand as they never disappoint. Great products and first-class customer service is their standard. I am a customer for life.

Love these!

Review by Tonya W. on 8 Jan 2022 review stating Love these!

I love the lemongrass body butter! After a long day, I look forward to settling down after a shower with the lemongrass scent, which reminds me of being in a high-end spa. It melts into the skin like true medicine—healing moisturizer is the perfect description for it. I wish they had larger jars.

Eczema Relief

Review by Gina D. on 27 May 2021 review stating Eczema Relief

I love the restoration salve and use it for my very dry skin. It provides tremendous relief from my eczema outbreaks. Very soothing and moisturizing.

Softness

Review by Valarie on 25 Sep 2021 review stating Softness

My daughter and I started using this soap after my niece raved about it, and now we want to rave about the creaminess of this soap. It exfoliates our face, leaving a clean, soft face. We have never gone wrong with any of their products. They create with love.

Healing and buttery soft

Review by MACK on 4 Dec 2020 review stating Healing and buttery soft

Four years ago, I had second-degree burns on my face and developed eczema on my face. Dry and peeling—was so unprofessional. So, I decided to buckle and create a regimen to heal my skin three years later. And after one year of consistent usage, my dark marks are faded, my skin is buttery soft, and eczema is rarely an issue and NEVER do I see dryness or peeling. A life saver and a confidence booster. Thanks Nature's Puree.

Thank You

It was a wonderful experience and an exciting challenge writing this book. I have been honored to take you on this journey of wellness through skin care with me. I thank you for taking the time to purchase and read this book. I hope your takeaway has inspired you to consider natural skin care products or has provided you with more knowledge of the world of natural skin care through the eyes of a physician.

Be well,
Dr. Christina
info@drchectordo.com
Follow me on IG, FB, and LinkedIn @drchectordo

Citations

1. Avail Dermatology. "History of Skincare Products." Avail Dermatology. rae/wp-content/uploads/2021/10/avail-epi-logo.png, September 17, 2020. https://availdermatology.com/history-of-skincare-products/.
2. Faccio, Greta. "Plant Complexity and Cosmetic Innovation." *iScience* 23, no. 8 (2020): 101358. https://doi.org/10.1016/j.isci.2020.101358.
3. Avail Dermatology. "History of Skincare Products." Avail Dermatology. rae/wp-content/uploads/2021/10/avail-epi-logo.png, September 17, 2020. https://availdermatology.com/history-of-skincare-products/.
4. Smithsonian. Cosmetics and Personal Care Products in the Medicine and Science Collections "Skin Care." https://www.si.edu/spotlight/health-hygiene-and-beauty/skin-care.
5. Smithsonian. Cosmetics and Personal Care Products in the Medicine and Science Collections "Skin Care." https://www.si.edu/spotlight/health-hygiene-and-beauty/skin-care.
6. Black History Heroes. "Annie Turnbo Malone: A Black Philanthropist and Entrepreneur." Black History Heroes. Accessed June 1, 2022. http://www.blackhistoryheroes.com/2010/10/annie-turnbo.html.
7. A Brief History of Black Beauty in the United States: Early 1900s. https://www.whatamud.com/blog/bhm20. February 9, 2020.
8. A&E Television Networks. "Madam C.J. Walker." Biography.com. A&E Television Networks, November 12, 2021. https://www.biography.com/inventor/madam-cj-walker.

9. Smithsonian. Cosmetics and Personal Care Products in the Medicine and Science Collections "Skin Care." https://www.si.edu/spotlight/health-hygiene-and-beauty/skin-care.

10. Library of Congress. "Business of Beauty: A Resource Guide: History of the Beauty Business." Research Guides, Library of Congress. Accessed June 1, 2022. https://guides.loc.gov/business-of-beauty/history.

11. Wallack, Grace. "Rethinking FDA's Regulation of Cosmetics." *Harvard Journal on Legislation* 56, no. 1 (Winter 2019): 311–339.

12. Wallack, Grace. "Rethinking FDA's Regulation of Cosmetics." *Harvard Journal on Legislation* 56, no. 1 (Winter 2019): 311–339.

13. Center for Food Safety and Applied Nutrition, US Food and Drug Administration. "Cosmetics & U.S. Law." US Food and Drug Administration. FDA. Accessed June 1, 2022. https://www.fda.gov/cosmetics/cosmetics-laws-regulations/cosmetics-us-law.

14. Center for Food Safety and Applied Nutrition, US Food and Drug Administration. "Cosmetics & U.S. Law." US Food and Drug Administration. FDA. Accessed June 1, 2022. https://www.fda.gov/cosmetics/cosmetics-laws-regulations/cosmetics-us-law.

15. Center for Food Safety and Applied Nutrition, US Food and Drug Administration. "Cosmetics & U.S. Law." US Food and Drug Administration. FDA. Accessed June 1, 2022. https://www.fda.gov/cosmetics/cosmetics-laws-regulations/cosmetics-us-law.

16. Center for Food Safety and Applied Nutrition, US Food and Drug Administration. "Cosmetics & U.S. Law." US Food and Drug Administration. FDA. Accessed June 1, 2022. https://www.fda.gov/cosmetics/cosmetics-laws-regulations/cosmetics-us-law.

17. Center for Food Safety and Applied Nutrition, US Food and Drug Administration. "FDA Authority over Cosmetics: How Cosmetics Are Not FDA-Approved." US Food and Drug Administration. FDA. Accessed June 1, 2022. https://www.fda.gov/cosmetics/cosmetics-laws-regulations/fda-

authority-over-cosmetics-how-cosmetics-are-not-fda-approved-are-fda-regulated.

18. Center for Food Safety and Applied Nutrition, US Food and Drug Administration. "FDA Authority over Cosmetics: How Cosmetics Are Not FDA-Approved." US Food and Drug Administration. FDA. Accessed June 1, 2022. https://www.fda.gov/cosmetics/cosmetics-laws-regulations/fda-authority-over-cosmetics-how-cosmetics-are-not-fda-approved-are-fda-regulated.

19. American Cleaning Institute. "Soap & Detergents History." American Cleaning Institute (ACI). Accessed June 20, 2022. https://www.cleaninginstitute.org/understanding-products/why-clean/soaps-detergents-history

20. American Cleaning Institute. "Soaps & Detergents History." The American Cleaning Institute (ACI). Accessed June 1, 2022. https://www.cleaninginstitute.org/understanding-products/why-clean/soaps-detergents-history.

21. American Cleaning Institute. "Soaps & Detergents History." The American Cleaning Institute (ACI). Accessed June 1, 2022. https://www.cleaninginstitute.org/understanding-products/why-clean/soaps-detergents-history.

22. US Consumer Product Safety Commission. "About Us." US Consumer Product Safety Commission. Accessed June 1, 2022. https://www.cpsc.gov/About-CPSC.

23. The National Law Review. "Natural Cosmetics: Products without a Clear Definition." The National Law Review. Accessed June 1, 2022. https://www.natlawreview.com/article/natural-cosmetics-products-without-clear-definition.

24. US Department of Agriculture. "USDA Certified Organic: Understanding the Basics." USDA Certified Organic: Understanding the Basics | Agricultural Marketing Service. Accessed June 1, 2022. https://www.ams.usda.gov/services/organic-certification/organic-basics.

25. Pandey, Amarendra, Jatana, Gurpoonam K., Sonthalia, Sidharth. *Cosmeceuticals*. Treasure Island: StatPearls Publishing, 2021.

26. Center for Food Safety and Applied Nutrition, US Food and Drug Administration. "Is It a Cosmetic, a Drug, or Both? (Or Is It Soap?)." US Food and Drug Administration. FDA. Accessed June 1, 2022. https://www.fda.gov/cosmetics/cosmetics-laws-regulations/it-cosmetic-drug-or-both-or-it-soap.

27. Dublin, (GLOBE NEWSWIRE) "Global Skincare Products Market (2021 to 2026) - Growth, Trends, COVID-19 Impact, and Forecasts". GlobeNewswire. April 19, 2021. Website. Accessed June 1, 2022. https://www.globenewswire.com/en/news-release/2021/04/19/2212301/28124/en/Global-Skincare-Products-Market-2021-to-2026-Growth-Trends-COVID-19-Impact-and-Forecasts.html#:~:text=The%20Global%20Skincare%20Products%20Market,the%20forecast%20period%202021%20%2D%202026.

28. The National Law Review. "Natural Cosmetics: Products without a Clear Definition." The National Law Review. Accessed June 1, 2022. https://www.natlawreview.com/article/natural-cosmetics-products-without-clear-definition.

29. Yousef, Hani. Alhajj, Mandy. Sharma, Sandeep. "Anatomy, Skin (Integument), Epidermis." In: *StatPearls*. Treasure Island: StatPearls Publishing, 2021.

30. Tabassum, Nahida, and Mariya Hamdani. "Plants Used to Treat Skin Diseases." *Pharmacognosy Reviews* 8, no. 15 (2014): 52. https://doi.org/10.4103/0973-7847.125531.

31. Poljšak, Borut, and Raja Dahmane. "Free Radicals and Extrinsic Skin Aging." *Dermatology Research and Practice* 2012 (2012): 1–4. https://doi.org/10.1155/2012/135206.

32. Sagbo, Idowu Jonas and Mbeng, Wilfred Otang. "Plants Used for Cosmetics in the Eastern Cape Province of South Africa: A Case Study of Skin Care." *Pharmacognosy Reviews* 12, no. 24 (2018): 139. https://doi.org/10.4103/phrev.phrev_9_18.

33. Emerald, Mila, Emerald, A., Emerald, L., and Kumar, Vikas. Perspective of Natural Products in Skincare. *Pharm Pharmacol Int J* *4*(3): 00072.

34. Environmental Working Group. "What Are Parabens, and Why Don't They Belong in Cosmetics?" Environmental Working Group. Accessed June 1, 2022. https://www.ewg.org/what-are-parabens.

35. Centers for Disease Control and Prevention. "Parabens Factsheet." Centers for Disease Control and Prevention, April 7, 2017. https://www.cdc.gov/biomonitoring/Parabens_FactSheet.html.

36. Wallack, Grace. "Rethinking FDA's Regulation of Cosmetics." *Harvard Journal on Legislation* 56, no. 1 (Winter 2019): 311–339.

37. Wallack, Grace. "Rethinking FDA's Regulation of Cosmetics." *Harvard Journal on Legislation* 56, no. 1 (Winter 2019): 311–339.

38. Malacoff, Julia. "Some Common Beauty Products Contain Formaldehyde - Why You Should Care." *Shape,* May 31, 2022. https://www.shape.com/lifestyle/beauty-style/common-beauty-products-formaldehyde-dangers.

39. Wallack, Grace. "Rethinking FDA's Regulation of Cosmetics." *Harvard Journal on Legislation* 56, no. 1 (Winter 2019): 311–339.

40. Wallack, Grace. "Rethinking FDA's Regulation of Cosmetics." *Harvard Journal on Legislation* 56, no. 1 (Winter 2019): 311–339.

41. Wallack, Grace. "Rethinking FDA's Regulation of Cosmetics." *Harvard Journal on Legislation* 56, no. 1 (Winter 2019): 311–339.

42. Wallack, Grace. "Rethinking FDA's Regulation of Cosmetics." *Harvard Journal on Legislation* 56, no. 1 (Winter 2019): 311–339.

43. Wallack, Grace. "Rethinking FDA's Regulation of Cosmetics." *Minion Pro Journal on Legislation* 56, no. 1 (Winter 2019): 311–339.

44. Wallack, Grace. "Rethinking FDA's Regulation of Cosmetics." *Minion Pro Journal on Legislation* 56, no. 1 (Winter 2019): 311–339.

45. Wallack, Grace. "Rethinking FDA's Regulation of Cosmetics." *Minion Pro Journal on Legislation* 56, no. 1 (Winter 2019): 311–339.

46. Wallack, Grace. "Rethinking FDA's Regulation of Cosmetics." *Minion Pro Journal on Legislation* 56, no. 1 (Winter 2019): 311–339.

47. Wallack, Grace. "Rethinking FDA's Regulation of Cosmetics." *Minion Pro Journal on Legislation* 56, no. 1 (Winter 2019): 311–339.

48. Wallack, Grace. "Rethinking FDA's Regulation of Cosmetics." *Minion Pro Journal on Legislation* 56, no. 1 (Winter 2019): 311–339.

49. Wallack, Grace. "Rethinking FDA's Regulation of Cosmetics." *Minion Pro Journal on Legislation* 56, no. 1 (Winter 2019): 311–339.

50. Wallack, Grace. "Rethinking FDA's Regulation of Cosmetics." *Minion Pro Journal on Legislation* 56, no. 1 (Winter 2019): 311–339.

51. Wallack, Grace. "Rethinking FDA's Regulation of Cosmetics." *Minion Pro Journal on Legislation* 56, no. 1 (Winter 2019): 311–339.

52. Wallack, Grace. "Rethinking FDA's Regulation of Cosmetics." *Minion Pro Journal on Legislation* 56, no. 1 (Winter 2019): 311–339.

53. Wallack, Grace. "Rethinking FDA's Regulation of Cosmetics." *Minion Pro Journal on Legislation* 56, no. 1 (Winter 2019): 311–339.

54. Safe Cosmetics. "International Laws." Safe Cosmetics. Accessed June 1, 2022. https://www.safecosmetics.org/get-the-facts/regulations/international-laws/.

55. Faber, Scott. EWG. The Toxic Twelve Chemicals and Contaminants in Cosmetics. May 5, 2020. Website. Accessed June 1, 2022. https://www.ewg.org/the-toxic-twelve-chemicals-and-contaminants-in-cosmetics.

56. California Legislative Information. "California Legislative Information." AB-2762 Cosmetic products: Safety. Accessed June 1, 2022. https://leginfo.legislature.ca.gov/faces/billTextClient.xhtml?bill_id=201920200AB2762.

57. Robin, Marci. "California Will Ban Two Dozen Ingredients from Beauty Products by 2025." *Allure*, October 1, 2020. https://www.allure.com/story/california-toxic-free-cosmetics-act-ban-chemicals-beauty-products.

58. Faccio, Greta. "Plant Complexity and Cosmetic Innovation." *iScience* 23, no. 8 (2020): 101358. https://doi.org/10.1016/j.isci.2020.101358.

59. Faccio, Greta. "Plant Complexity and Cosmetic Innovation." *iScience* 23, no. 8 (2020): 101358. https://doi.org/10.1016/j.isci.2020.101358.

60. US Department of Agriculture. "USDA Certified Organic: Understanding the Basics." USDA Certified Organic: Understanding the Basics | Agricultural Marketing Service. Accessed June 1, 2022. https://www.ams.usda.gov/services/organic-certification/organic-basics.

61. Beauchamp, Tom L., DeGrazia, David, and Akhtar, Aysha. The Flaws and Human Harms of Animal Experimentation. *Camb Q Healthc Ethics. 24*(4): 407–419. 2015.

62. Munoz, Sophie N. "Natural Ingredients, Are Not Always Better in Skincare." *StudyBreaks.* February 27, 2021. Website. Accessed June 23, 2022. https://studybreaks.com/thoughts/natural-vs-synthetic-skincare/.

63. Munoz, Sophie N. "Natural Ingredients Are Not Always Better in Skincare." *StudyBreaks.* February 27, 2021. Website. Accessed June 23, 2022. https://studybreaks.com/thoughts/natural-vs-synthetic-skincare/.

64. Wise, Lauren A., Palmer, Julie R., Reich, David, Cozier, Yvette C., and Rosenberg, Lynn. "Hair Relaxer Use and Risk of Uterine Leiomyomata in African-American Women." *American Journal of Epidemiology* 175, no. 5 (2012): 432–40. https://doi.org/10.1093/aje/kwr351.

65. Wallack, Grace. "Rethinking FDA's Regulation of Cosmetics." *Harvard Journal on Legislation* 56, no. 1 (Winter 2019): 311–339.

66. Kumar, Vikas. "Perspective of Natural Products in Skincare." *Pharmacy & Pharmacology International Journal* 4, no. 3 (2016). https://doi.org/10.15406/ppij.2016.04.00072.

67. Kumar, Vikas. "Perspective of Natural Products in Skincare." *Pharmacy & Pharmacology International Journal* 4, no. 3 (2016). https://doi.org/10.15406/ppij.2016.04.00072.

68. Sethi, Anisha, Kaur, Tejinder, Malhotra, S.K.M., and Gambhir, M.L. "Moisturizers: The Slippery Road." *Indian Journal of Dermatology* 61, no. 3 (2016): 279. https://doi.org/10.4103/0019-5154.182427.

69. Sethi, Anisha, Kaur, Tejinder, Malhotra, S.K.M., and Gambhir, M.L. "Moisturizers: The Slippery Road." *Indian Journal of Dermatology* 61, no. 3 (2016): 279. https://doi.org/10.4103/0019-5154.182427.

70. Sethi, Anisha, Kaur, Tejinder, Malhotra, S.K.M., and Gambhir, M.L. "Moisturizers: The Slippery Road." *Indian Journal of Dermatology* 61, no. 3 (2016): 279. https://doi.org/10.4103/0019-5154.182427.

71. Lin, Tzu-Kai, Zhong, Lily, and Santiago, Juan. "Anti-Inflammatory and Skin Barrier Repair Effects of Topical Application of Some Plant Oils." *International Journal of Molecular Sciences* 19, no. 1 (2017): 70. https://doi.org/10.3390/ijms19010070.

72. Lin, Tzu-Kai, Zhong, Lily, and Santiago, Juan. "Anti-Inflammatory and Skin Barrier Repair Effects of Topical Application of Some Plant Oils." *International Journal of Molecular Sciences* 19, no. 1 (2017): 70. https://doi.org/10.3390/ijms19010070.

73. Lin, Tzu-Kai, Zhong, Lily, and Santiago, Juan. "Anti-Inflammatory and Skin Barrier Repair Effects of Topical Application of Some Plant Oils." *International Journal of Molecular Sciences* 19, no. 1 (2017): 70. https://doi.org/10.3390/ijms19010070.

74. Lin, Tzu-Kai, Zhong, Lily, and Santiago, Juan. "Anti-Inflammatory and Skin Barrier Repair Effects of Topical Application of Some

Plant Oils." *International Journal of Molecular Sciences* 19, no. 1 (2017): 70. https://doi.org/10.3390/ijms19010070.

75. Lin, Tzu-Kai, Zhong, Lily, and Santiago, Juan. "Anti-Inflammatory and Skin Barrier Repair Effects of Topical Application of Some Plant Oils." *International Journal of Molecular Sciences* 19, no. 1 (2017): 70. https://doi.org/10.3390/ijms19010070.

76. Lin, Tzu-Kai, Zhong, Lily, and Santiago, Juan. "Anti-Inflammatory and Skin Barrier Repair Effects of Topical Application of Some Plant Oils." *International Journal of Molecular Sciences* 19, no. 1 (2017): 70. https://doi.org/10.3390/ijms19010070.

77. Lin, Tzu-Kai, Zhong, Lily, and Santiago, Juan. "Anti-Inflammatory and Skin Barrier Repair Effects of Topical Application of Some Plant Oils." *International Journal of Molecular Sciences* 19, no. 1 (2017): 70. https://doi.org/10.3390/ijms19010070.

78. Lin, Tzu-Kai, Zhong, Lily, and Santiago, Juan. "Anti-Inflammatory and Skin Barrier Repair Effects of Topical Application of Some Plant Oils." *International Journal of Molecular Sciences* 19, no. 1 (2017): 70. https://doi.org/10.3390/ijms19010070.

79. Woolf, Allan, Wong, Marie, Eyres, Laurence, Mcghie, Tony. "Avocado Oil." *Gourmet and Health-Promoting Specialty Oils*. 2009. pp.73–125.

80. Lin, Tzu-Kai, Zhong, Lily, and Santiago, Juan. "Anti-Inflammatory and Skin Barrier Repair Effects of Topical Application of Some Plant Oils." *International Journal of Molecular Sciences* 19, no. 1 (2017): 70. https://doi.org/10.3390/ijms19010070.

81. Femenia, A. "High-Value Co-Products from Plant Foods: Cosmetics and Pharmaceuticals." *Handbook of Waste Management and Co-Product Recovery in Food Processing* 1 (2007): 470–501. https://doi.org/10.1533/9781845692520.4.470.

82. Femenia, A. "High-Value Co-Products from Plant Foods: Cosmetics and Pharmaceuticals." *Handbook of Waste Management and*

Co-Product Recovery in Food Processing 1 (2007): 470–501. https://doi.org/10.1533/9781845692520.4.470.

83. Lin, Tzu-Kai, Zhong, Lily, and Santiago, Juan. "Anti-Inflammatory and Skin Barrier Repair Effects of Topical Application of Some Plant Oils." *International Journal of Molecular Sciences* 19, no. 1 (2017): 70. https://doi.org/10.3390/ijms19010070.
84. Lin, Tzu-Kai, Zhong, Lily, and Santiago, Juan. "Anti-Inflammatory and Skin Barrier Repair Effects of Topical Application of Some Plant Oils." *International Journal of Molecular Sciences* 19, no. 1 (2017): 70. https://doi.org/10.3390/ijms19010070.
85. Ahmad, Zeeshan. "The Uses and Properties of Almond Oil." *Complementary Therapies in Clinical Practice* 16, no. 1 (2010): 10–12. https://doi.org/10.1016/j.ctcp.2009.06.015.
86. Lin, Tzu-Kai, Zhong, Lily, and Santiago, Juan. "Anti-Inflammatory and Skin Barrier Repair Effects of Topical Application of Some Plant Oils." *International Journal of Molecular Sciences* 19, no. 1 (2017): 70. https://doi.org/10.3390/ijms19010070.
87. Srivastava, Janmejai K., Shankar, Eswar, and Gupta, Sanjay. "Chamomile: A Herbal Medicine of the Past with a Bright Future (Review)." *Molecular Medicine Reports* 3, no. 6 (2010). https://doi.org/10.3892/mmr.2010.377.
88. Srivastava, Janmejai K., Shankar, Eswar, and Gupta, Sanjay. "Chamomile: A Herbal Medicine of the Past with a Bright Future (Review)." *Molecular Medicine Reports* 3, no. 6 (2010). https://doi.org/10.3892/mmr.2010.377.
89. Srivastava, Janmejai K., Shankar, Eswar, and Gupta, Sanjay. "Chamomile: A Herbal Medicine of the Past with a Bright Future (Review)." *Molecular Medicine Reports* 3, no. 6 (2010). https://doi.org/10.3892/mmr.2010.377.
90. Lin, Tzu-Kai, Zhong, Lily, and Santiago, Juan. "Anti-Inflammatory and Skin Barrier Repair Effects of Topical Application of Some

Plant Oils." *International Journal of Molecular Sciences* 19, no. 1 (2017): 70. https://doi.org/10.3390/ijms19010070.

91. Lin, Tzu-Kai, Zhong, Lily, and Santiago, Juan. "Anti-Inflammatory and Skin Barrier Repair Effects of Topical Application of Some Plant Oils." *International Journal of Molecular Sciences* 19, no. 1 (2017): 70. https://doi.org/10.3390/ijms19010070.
92. Israel, Malachi Oluwaseyi. "Effects of Topical and Dietary Use of Shea Butter on Animals." *American Journal of Life Sciences* 2, no. 5 (2014): 303. https://doi.org/10.11648/j.ajls.20140205.18.
93. Israel, Malachi Oluwaseyi. "Effects of Topical and Dietary Use of Shea Butter on Animals." *American Journal of Life Sciences* 2, no. 5 (2014): 303. https://doi.org/10.11648/j.ajls.20140205.18.
94. Lin, Tzu-Kai, Zhong, Lily, and Santiago, Juan. "Anti-Inflammatory and Skin Barrier Repair Effects of Topical Application of Some Plant Oils." *International Journal of Molecular Sciences* 19, no. 1 (2017): 70. https://doi.org/10.3390/ijms19010070.
95. Lin, Tzu-Kai, Zhong, Lily, and Santiago, Juan. "Anti-Inflammatory and Skin Barrier Repair Effects of Topical Application of Some Plant Oils." *International Journal of Molecular Sciences* 19, no. 1 (2017): 70. https://doi.org/10.3390/ijms19010070.
96. Lin, Tzu-Kai, Zhong, Lily, and Santiago, Juan. "Anti-Inflammatory and Skin Barrier Repair Effects of Topical Application of Some Plant Oils." *International Journal of Molecular Sciences* 19, no. 1 (2017): 70. https://doi.org/10.3390/ijms19010070.
97. Stoia, Mihaela and Oancea, Simona. "Selected Evidence-Based Health Benefits of Topically Applied Sunflower Oil." *Applied Science Reports 10*(1). 2015. https://doi.org/10.15192/pscp.asr.2015.10.1.4549.
98. Lin, Tzu-Kai, Zhong, Lily, and Santiago, Juan. "Anti-Inflammatory and Skin Barrier Repair Effects of Topical Application of Some Plant Oils." *International Journal of Molecular Sciences* 19, no. 1 (2017): 70. https://doi.org/10.3390/ijms19010070.

99. Lin, Tzu-Kai, Zhong, Lily, and Santiago, Juan. "Anti-Inflammatory and Skin Barrier Repair Effects of Topical Application of Some Plant Oils." *International Journal of Molecular Sciences* 19, no. 1 (2017): 70. https://doi.org/10.3390/ijms19010070.

100. Lin, Tzu-Kai, Zhong, Lily, and Santiago, Juan. "Anti-Inflammatory and Skin Barrier Repair Effects of Topical Application of Some Plant Oils." *International Journal of Molecular Sciences* 19, no. 1 (2017): 70. https://doi.org/10.3390/ijms19010070.

101. https://doi.org/10.3390/ijms19010070.

102. Lin, Tzu-Kai, Zhong, Lily, and Santiago, Juan. "Anti-Inflammatory and Skin Barrier Repair Effects of Topical Application of Some Plant Oils." *International Journal of Molecular Sciences* 19, no. 1 (2017): 70. https://doi.org/10.3390/ijms19010070.

103. Lin, Tzu-Kai, Zhong, Lily, and Santiago, Juan. "Anti-Inflammatory and Skin Barrier Repair Effects of Topical Application of Some Plant Oils." *International Journal of Molecular Sciences* 19, no. 1 (2017): 70. https://doi.org/10.3390/ijms19010070.

104. Lin, Tzu-Kai, Zhong, Lily, and Santiago, Juan. "Anti-Inflammatory and Skin Barrier Repair Effects of Topical Application of Some Plant Oils." *International Journal of Molecular Sciences* 19, no. 1 (2017): 70. https://doi.org/10.3390/ijms19010070.

105. Lin, Tzu-Kai, Zhong, Lily, and Santiago, Juan. "Anti-Inflammatory and Skin Barrier Repair Effects of Topical Application of Some Plant Oils." *International Journal of Molecular Sciences* 19, no. 1 (2017): 70. https://doi.org/10.3390/ijms19010070.

106. Lin, Tzu-Kai, Zhong, Lily, and Santiago, Juan. "Anti-Inflammatory and Skin Barrier Repair Effects of Topical Application of Some Plant Oils." *International Journal of Molecular Sciences* 19, no. 1 (2017): 70. https://doi.org/10.3390/ijms19010070.

107. Lin, Tzu-Kai, Zhong, Lily, and Santiago, Juan. "Anti-Inflammatory and Skin Barrier Repair Effects of Topical Application of Some

Plant Oils." *International Journal of Molecular Sciences* 19, no. 1 (2017): 70. https://doi.org/10.3390/ijms19010070.

108. Lin, Tzu-Kai, Zhong, Lily, and Santiago, Juan. "Anti-Inflammatory and Skin Barrier Repair Effects of Topical Application of Some Plant Oils." *International Journal of Molecular Sciences* 19, no. 1 (2017): 70. https://doi.org/10.3390/ijms19010070.

109. Faccio, Greta. "Plant Complexity and Cosmetic Innovation." *iScience* 23, no. 8 (2020): 101358. https://doi.org/10.1016/j.isci.2020.101358.

110. Lin, Tzu-Kai, Zhong, Lily, and Santiago, Juan. "Anti-Inflammatory and Skin Barrier Repair Effects of Topical Application of Some Plant Oils." *International Journal of Molecular Sciences* 19, no. 1 (2017): 70. https://doi.org/10.3390/ijms19010070.

111. Lin, Tzu-Kai, Zhong, Lily, and Santiago, Juan. "Anti-Inflammatory and Skin Barrier Repair Effects of Topical Application of Some Plant Oils." *International Journal of Molecular Sciences* 19, no. 1 (2017): 70. https://doi.org/10.3390/ijms19010070.

112. Lin, Tzu-Kai, Zhong, Lily, and Santiago, Juan. "Anti-Inflammatory and Skin Barrier Repair Effects of Topical Application of Some Plant Oils." *International Journal of Molecular Sciences* 19, no. 1 (2017): 70. https://doi.org/10.3390/ijms19010070.

113. Lin, Tzu-Kai, Zhong, Lily, and Santiago, Juan. "Anti-Inflammatory and Skin Barrier Repair Effects of Topical Application of Some Plant Oils." *International Journal of Molecular Sciences* 19, no. 1 (2017): 70. https://doi.org/10.3390/ijms19010070.

114. Lin, Tzu-Kai, Zhong, Lily, and Santiago, Juan. "Anti-Inflammatory and Skin Barrier Repair Effects of Topical Application of Some Plant Oils." *International Journal of Molecular Sciences* 19, no. 1 (2017): 70. https://doi.org/10.3390/ijms19010070.

115. Lin, Tzu-Kai, Zhong, Lily, and Santiago, Juan. "Anti-Inflammatory and Skin Barrier Repair Effects of Topical Application of Some

Plant Oils." *International Journal of Molecular Sciences* 19, no. 1 (2017): 70. https://doi.org/10.3390/ijms19010070.

116. Lin, Tzu-Kai, Zhong, Lily, and Santiago, Juan. "Anti-Inflammatory and Skin Barrier Repair Effects of Topical Application of Some Plant Oils." *International Journal of Molecular Sciences* 19, no. 1 (2017): 70. https://doi.org/10.3390/ijms19010070.

117. Lin, Tzu-Kai, Zhong, Lily, and Santiago, Juan. "Anti-Inflammatory and Skin Barrier Repair Effects of Topical Application of Some Plant Oils." *International Journal of Molecular Sciences* 19, no. 1 (2017): 70. https://doi.org/10.3390/ijms19010070.

118. Lin, Tzu-Kai, Zhong, Lily, and Santiago, Juan. "Anti-Inflammatory and Skin Barrier Repair Effects of Topical Application of Some Plant Oils." *International Journal of Molecular Sciences* 19, no. 1 (2017): 70. https://doi.org/10.3390/ijms19010070.

119. Lin, Tzu-Kai, Zhong, Lily, and Santiago, Juan. "Anti-Inflammatory and Skin Barrier Repair Effects of Topical Application of Some Plant Oils." *International Journal of Molecular Sciences* 19, no. 1 (2017): 70. https://doi.org/10.3390/ijms19010070.

120. Rampáčková, Eliška, Göttingerová, Martina, Gála, Pavel, Kiss, Tomáš, Ercisli, Sezai, and Nečas, Tomáš. "Evaluation of Protein and Antioxidant Content in Apricot Kernels as a Sustainable Additional Source of Nutrition." *Sustainability* 13, no. 9 (2021): 4742. https://doi.org/10.3390/su13094742.

121. Rampáčková, Eliška, Göttingerová, Martina, Gála, Pavel, Kiss, Tomáš, Ercisli, Sezai, and Nečas, Tomáš. "Evaluation of Protein and Antioxidant Content in Apricot Kernels as a Sustainable Additional Source of Nutrition." *Sustainability* 13, no. 9 (2021): 4742. https://doi.org/10.3390/su13094742.

122. Lin, Tzu-Kai, Zhong, Lily, and Santiago, Juan. "Anti-Inflammatory and Skin Barrier Repair Effects of Topical Application of Some Plant Oils." *International Journal of Molecular Sciences* 19, no. 1 (2017): 70. https://doi.org/10.3390/ijms19010070.

123. Silva, Diva, Salvador Ferreira, Marta, Manuel Sousa-Lobo, José, Cruz, Maria Teresa, and Filipa Almeida, Isabel. "Anti-Inflammatory Activity of Calendula Officinalis L. Flower Extract." *Cosmetics* 8, no. 2 (2021): 31. https://doi.org/10.3390/cosmetics8020031.

124. Tabassum, Nahida and Hamdani, Mariya. "Plants Used to Treat Skin Diseases." *Pharmacognosy Reviews* 8, no. 15 (2014): 52. https://doi.org/10.4103/0973-7847.125531.

125. Tabassum, Nahida and Hamdani, Mariya. "Plants Used to Treat Skin Diseases." *Pharmacognosy Reviews* 8, no. 15 (2014): 52. https://doi.org/10.4103/0973-7847.125531.

126. Surjushe, Amar, Vasani, Resham, and Saple, DG. "Aloe Vera: A Short Review." *Indian Journal of Dermatology* 53, no. 4 (2008): 163. https://doi.org/10.4103/0019-5154.44785.

127. Surjushe, Amar, Vasani, Resham, and Saple, DG. "Aloe Vera: A Short Review." *Indian Journal of Dermatology* 53, no. 4 (2008): 163. https://doi.org/10.4103/0019-5154.44785.

128. Surjushe, Amar, Vasani, Resham, and Saple, DG. "Aloe Vera: A Short Review." *Indian Journal of Dermatology* 53, no. 4 (2008): 163. https://doi.org/10.4103/0019-5154.44785.

129. Surjushe, Amar, Vasani, Resham, and Saple, DG. "Aloe Vera: A Short Review." *Indian Journal of Dermatology* 53, no. 4 (2008): 163. https://doi.org/10.4103/0019-5154.44785.

130. Dearie, KJ. "Product Disclaimer: Examples & Guide." Termly, May 12, 2022. https://termly.io/resources/articles/product-disclaimer/.

131. OB-GYN, Moreland. "Essential Oils and Pregnancy Safety." Moreland OB-GYN Leading Women to Better Health. 2019. https://www.morelandobgyn.com/blog/essential-oils-and-pregnancy-safety.

About the Author

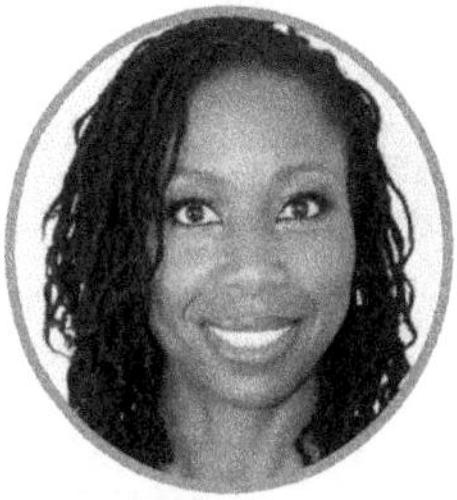

Dr. Christina Hector, DO, is a board-certified sports medicine and family medicine physician. She is the founder of Nature's Purée LLC, whose mission is to change the standard of skin care to where the leading skin care products used by families are made with natural ingredients.

Born and raised in Brooklyn, NY, Dr. Hector earned her bachelor of science from Northeastern University and her doctorate of osteopathic medicine from the University of Medicine and Dentistry of New Jersey. She completed her family medicine residency at Crozer Keystone Hospital and her primary care sports medicine fellowship at Atlantic Sports Health. She is also the co-founder of Onyx Direct Care, a micro-concierge practice geared at providing well-balanced, comprehensive musculoskeletal care for patients.

Dr. Hector is a proud wife and mother of three children. In her free time, she enjoys exercising, DIY projects, and spending time with her family.

To connect, follow Nature's Purée on Instagram, Facebook, and Pinterest @naturespuree. For additional information contact us at orders@naturespuree.com

CPSIA information can be obtained
at www.ICGtesting.com
Printed in the USA
BVHW052335020223
657810BV00023B/131

9 781644 845950